Further praise for *Life After a Partner's Suicide Attempt*

"When a person attempts suicide, the world often falls in around their partners and families. Surprisingly, this book is the first scholarly attempt to let partners speak about how that traumatic event impacted them. The stories told here reveal an often life-altering maelstrom of relief, grief, disbelief, doubt, care, exhaustion, exasperation, worry, loneliness, ongoing fear and roller-coaster love that requires huge resilience to navigate. Yet there is hope and help as Dr. McGivern's seminal work convincingly charts – opening up a neglected landscape for recognition and discussion."
Dr. Mary McAleese, former President of Ireland and Professor of Children, Law & Religion, University of Glasgow

"McGivern has written an impactful book for the millions who experience the trauma of being partnered with someone surviving a suicide attempt. Some relationships are irrevocably damaged, while for others, post-traumatic growth occurs. The inspiration McGivern provides enhances the chances of suffering becoming a transformative experience for both partners and is, therefore, a very important contribution to the field."
Linda Bloom, LCSW, Psychotherapist at Bloomwork in California and co-author of *101 Things I Wish I Knew When I Got Married: Simple Lessons to Make Love Last*

"This inspiring book explores the traumatic impact of a partner's attempted suicide through the intimate stories of those who have experienced this life changing event. Dr. McGivern brings together relevant theoretical perspectives, clinical models and practical strategies to deepen our understanding and to support this neglected population, often considered only in the shadow role of caregiver. These anguished first-hand accounts convey the shocking betrayal of trust, and complex adjustment required to integrate adverse and positive transformative processes. The book shines a powerful light, showing the potential benefits for both partners of incorporating a systemic approach in the quest for relational healing, growth and hope."
Diana Sands PhD, Director, Centre for Intense Grief Therapy, Sydney, Australia

"By faithfully narrating the stories of the partners of those who have attempted suicide in their own words, *Life After a Partner's Suicide Attempt* plays an important role in shining a light on and increasing awareness and understanding of their lived experience, and identifies ways by which to better support them in their own journey towards recovery."
Eddie Ward, HSE Resource Officer for Suicide Prevention, Louth/Meath

Life
after a
partner's
suicide
attempt

Life
after a
partner's
suicide
attempt

Francis McGivern

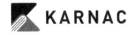 KARNAC

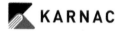

KARNAC

First published in 2021 by Karnac Books, an imprint of Confer Ltd.

www.confer.uk.com

Registered office:
Brody House, Strype Street, London E1 7LQ

1 3 5 7 9 10 8 6 4 2

British Library Cataloguing in Publication Data
A catalogue record for this book is available from the British Library.

ISBN: 978-1-913494-34-6 (paperback)
ISBN: 978-1-913494-35-3 (ebook)

Typeset by Bespoke Publishing Ltd
Printed in the UK by Ashford Colour Press

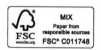

Contents

List of Figures

Acknowledgements

First and foremost, I extend my heartfelt appreciation to the individuals who participated in this research. Your courage and generosity are abundant, and your insights will no doubt positively touch countless others around the world. Thank you to my wife and children for your patience when I was lost in my laptop. My thanks to Ms Sofie Owens (MA Literary Studies, Queen's University Belfast) who provided editorial guidance with parts of the manuscript. Thank you to Ms. Catherine Butterly, MA Counselling Coordinator, Webster University, Geneva, Switzerland who first introduced me to ambiguous loss theory. Thanks also to Ms Sheena McKenna, psychotherapist and former journalist, who proofread final drafts of the manuscript.

This book is based on original research conducted through Dublin City University, Dublin, Ireland.

Preface

Part I of this book provides an insight into how a chance encounter in my role as a counselling psychologist and psychotherapist piqued my interest in pursuing research in this never before identified area of suicidology. It then delves directly into in-depth interviews with partners of individuals who attempted suicide. These accounts are first-hand and uncensored, thereby allowing partners to portray the transformative impact of the attempt on their lives in an articulate and highly emotional way, and with minimal need for analysis on my part. Readers who may have lived through a similar event will probably strongly identify with these accounts, and for many it may feel like acknowledgement of their lived experience, perhaps for the first time ever. Readers who have an interest in this area either casual or professional, are sure to develop greater empathy for those who have lived through this event as a result.

Part II begins with an assessment of how potentially far-reaching the social impact of a suicide attempt may be, beyond the suicide attempter him or herself. It then provides an overview of previous research in this area from as far back as the early 1960s and, in so doing, highlight the stark lack of interest in the personal impact on partners beyond their role as caregiver. Based on insights gathered from the interviews in Part I, it then offers mental health and medical professionals, and partners themselves, not only a means of making sense of their experience but also a roadmap towards their recovery following their loved one's suicide attempt. Recommendations for practice and policy are offered, concluding with implications for future research.

PART I

GIVING VOICE TO PARTNERS

CHAPTER I

The inspiration for this book: a psychotherapy session like no other

'He has put it firmly in the past, [but] it's never in the past for me. It comes across on the radio interviews you hear, it comes across on the news, it comes every time you hear of a suicide, every time I hear of a missing person. It never goes away. Never *ever* goes away ... And I don't think I ever will get over it ... It's happened, I can't undo it. He apologized, he regrets it ...[but] our relationship was never the same again, never ... and I really don't think it ever will be because I know *I'm* not the same person I was.' (extract from interview)

From the moment I heard these words uttered, I knew immediately that this woman had captured, in one breath, so much of what people live through following a partner's suicide attempt. This includes the trauma of the experience, the transformative impact on their view of themselves, the world and their relationship, and the permanency of all of this. What's more, this same woman also noticed that after the experience of her partner's suicide attempt, 'Very few people, *very* few people ever said, "How are you?"'. While attention from medical and mental health professionals as well as family members is appropriately paid to the individual who has made an attempt on their life in order to ensure their safety and comfort, the focus of this book is to shine a light on the personal experience of those closest to that person, namely their partner. Placing the focus firmly on the personal impact on partners is in no way intended to minimize or discount the gravity of the suicide attempter's situation. Rather, it is intended to broaden the knowledge base of the wider impact of this event to *include* partners.

The language and terminology applied to this sensitive area has historically been problematic and confusing. However, a large-scale anonymous online survey conducted in 2019, in which people affected in some way by suicide were asked to rate their perceived acceptability of terms related to suicidal behaviour (Padmanathan *et al.*, 2019), revealed that 'attempted suicide' above all other terms (including 'non-fatal self-harm' and 'suicidal gesture'), was deemed most acceptable. I chose to use the term 'attempted suicide' both in reverence to this finding and to be clear that there has been no fatality. Therefore, the term 'suicide attempt', which is at times used interchangeably with 'attempted suicide' throughout, shall be defined here as:

A serious self-harming event with a clear intention of death but with no such outcome.

There can be variation in how the individual engaging in suicidal behaviour, their partners, as well as healthcare professionals, interpret the actual level of intent regarding a suicidal act. Whether the intention was to break free from unbearable distress or a resolute desire to die, it is worth noting that relatives 'may intuitively interpret an act of suicidal behaviour far worse than the individual performing the act' (Juel, Berring, Hybholt, Erlangsen, Larsen and Buus, 2020, p. 2). This finding in itself speaks to the extent to which relatives can potentially be profoundly impacted by an individual's suicide attempt regardless of the actual intention behind the behaviour.

If you are reading this book, you are likely to be someone who loves or has loved a person who has attempted suicide. The book is aimed specifically towards partners of individuals who have attempted suicide. In any couple relationship both individuals can be ascribed the term 'partner'. I have endeavoured, however, to be as clear as possible in my writing so the reader can differentiate between both parties, that is, the partner who attempts suicide and the partner in a relationship with the attempter.

The firsthand accounts from partners, however, should also resonate with 'significant others'. Significant others would tend to be anyone who features in the suicide attempter's life in a meaningful way, including parents, adult children, siblings, friends, as well as other non-relatives. Alternatively, you may be a medical or mental health professional who is supporting those who love or have loved someone who has experienced a suicide attempt. Whether you are a partner, a significant other or a health professional, you will be familiar with the moral and cultural expectation to rally around others in critical need of care and attention.

Altruism or putting the welfare of others before our own is a trait that has been strongly reinforced in our culture from an early age. This response is clear to see, and some may say justified, in situations in which someone's life is in danger due to the threat of suicide or an attempted suicide. Society quickly rallies around the suicide attempters: first responders, emergency medical technicians, doctors, nurses, priests, other professionals, and significant others. The individual's life partner (spouse or long-term partner) usually becomes the *most* significant of significant others and the 'baton' in this 'relay' is swiftly handed over to them. In the immediate aftermath of a suicide attempt, emphasis is understandably placed on monitoring the individual at risk and developing ways of keeping them physically safe.

Partners are strongly encouraged from the outset, by medical personnel and the individual's family alike, to *manage* this crisis to keep the suicide attempter safe. In my clinical experience, however, I have found that the partner's emotional response to want to take care of the suicide attempter can be significantly overshadowed by so many hidden aspects of the experience including their own mixed feelings about the event, the pressure that is placed on them in their role as partner, and the changes that occur within the relationship after the attempt. In fact, the will to care can actually be overshadowed by the trauma of the event itself. There are so many complex aspects to this trauma, all of which will be highlighted in the chapters that follow. Of all the potential crises to which partnerships can be exposed, this crisis is one in which the partner of the suicide attempter is *least* likely to feel justified and supported in looking after themselves. The partner's complex response to the individual's suicide attempt is often not recognized by others and is, therefore, sidelined by virtually everyone they encounter.

A number of years ago, I began working with a woman who sought out psychotherapeutic support with me approximately six months after her husband had attempted suicide. It was clear from our very first session together that she was sharing thoughts and feelings, and a perspective, that had rarely, if ever, been shared before. It was a psychotherapy session like no other. During it, she described having almost immediately been dubbed 'chief caregiver' to her husband following his attempt by both hospital staff and family members. Her own difficult journey that arose as a result of his attempt was made all the more complicated by the very mixed feelings she now had about him and what he had done. She felt that her perspective was neither recognized nor accepted by those around her. My encounter with this woman made me confront the expectation, both my own and that of society, that people are always inherently motivated to care for others. This applies to spouses, in particular, who end up in a very vulnerable position. All of this roused my interest in looking beyond the role of caregiver to explore the *personal* experience of individuals who have encountered a partner's suicide attempt.

Imagine a motorway with a fast and slow lane. The suicide attempter wants to move quickly into the fast lane of recovery without looking back. Family members, however, remain in the slow lane. They are fearful of moving forward too quickly and, at the same time, reluctant to let go of the past. This particular client, therefore, provided the impetus for this book which aims, for the first time, to shine a light on the personal experience of partners whose lives are forever transformed in the wake of their loved one's suicide attempt. In doing so, it highlights the fundamental need for them to pay attention to their own mental health as they navigate this uncharted territory. It is, in effect, an opportunity to ask that question that was seldom, if ever, asked: 'How are you?' The question I wanted to explore in this book, 'What is the personal impact of a suicide attempt on partners?', brought me on an unbelievable journey during which I met inspirational people whose stories I want to share with you here.

The individuals you are about to meet in the pages that follow are those who were both brave enough and kind enough to participate in an interview with me as part of a study I was doing into the personal impact of an attempted suicide on partners. A total of five separate in-depth interviews were conducted and later analysed. This may at first seem like a small number of individuals. However, the emphasis was about capturing in great detail and depth their personal lived experience rather than getting a less informative snapshot of generic symptoms from a large number of people.

They were identified as potential participants in the study through various means but primarily through family doctors. Since these doctors were thought to typically have a long-established relationship with their patients that was built on trust, they were best placed to determine suitable candidates for such a sensitive study. Alternative sources of recruitment included mental health organizations such as *Suicide or*

Survive (an Irish charity that supports those recovering from a suicide attempt) and *AWARE* (another Irish charity that provides support for individuals experiencing depression or bipolar disorder).

The people to whom I wanted to talk about this experience did not necessarily have to be married to the person who attempted suicide because I believed this phenomenon applied to any individual who recognized their relationship as an *established, meaningful* one. Consequently, I made it clear from the outset that I wanted to hear from 'partners' of those who attempted suicide, which included spouse, common-law spouse, and long-term partner. Those who expressed an interest in taking part in the research and who also proved suitable for the study all had important things in common. They were all over eighteen years of age, they were all in a meaningful relationship, and their partners had made a first-time, non-fatal suicide attempt. This suicide attempt had occurred a *minimum* of six months before participation. This sensitive timeline was chosen in order to respect the enormity of the impact on interview participants so as not to retraumatize them in any way. In fact, the average time since their partner's attempted suicide at interview was much longer than anticipated, which meant they felt much more comfortable in providing an incredibly rich insight into both the personal impact on them and their relationship since the event.

Figure 1 aims to provide a visual depiction of the main themes that surfaced following the analysis of all five interviews, thereby aiding the reader in conceptualizing the partner's lived experience. It may prove useful to refer back to Figure 1 intermittently as a visual means of positioning Chapters 2, 3, and 4 within the context of the analysis.

Participants described their experience using stark imagery like wanting to 'scream from the mountain tops' and metaphors such as their 'whole world shifting on its axis', a 'show-stopper' and referenced it as an event of 'monumental' proportions. They interpreted the suicide attempt as traumatic and its aftermath as an act of survival for them. However, they also felt that the experience triggered a longer-term effect of increased personal strength as well as having the effect of enhancing their relationships with others. It is important to note that enhancement of relationships did not necessarily occur in the relationship with the suicide attempter as we might have assumed. It is normal within the lifespan of any long-term relationship to experience fluctuation, or what might more commonly be known as 'ups and downs'. It will be apparent as you become acquainted with each interview participant that these couples' experiences are no different to any other long-term relationship in this respect. The focus of this book is to elucidate the personal impact of a suicide attempt on partners and part of this exploration, for some, entailed their personal perception of the quality and status of their relationship prior to, and in the aftermath of, the attempt. Altogether, their stories reflect the importance, scale, and far-reaching consequences of this event for them.

The main theme '"I'm not the same person I was": transformations for better, for worse', captures the paradox that was the lived experience of all participants following the attempted suicide of their partners. 'For better, for worse' is

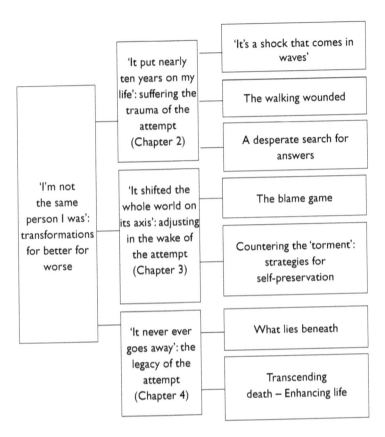

Figure 1 *Main themes emerging from analysis of interviews*

also a reference to the marriage vows traditionally undertaken by couples as a mark of their mutual commitment to the relationship.

The centre of Figure 1 represents three key subthemes that were also identified. The first theme '"It put nearly ten years on my life": suffering the trauma of the attempt' articulates the sheer force of the impact on participants.

Both at the time of their partners' suicide attempts and in the early aftermath, they faced complex struggles to process the shock to which they were exposed and all that came with it, including emotional upheaval and sensory overload, the acknowledgement of hurt in the midst of practical obligations, and a barrage of unanswered questions.

The second theme entitled '"It shifted the whole world on its axis": adjusting in the wake of the attempt' reflects the harrowing journey taken by participants as they came to terms with these permanently life-changing events. An unavoidable part of this journey involved thrashing out whom or what was responsible for their partners trying to kill themselves. It was an uncomfortable but necessary process to go through in order to move forward. Participants began questioning their ability to withstand the torment that the situation had created for them. This torment caused them to develop various means of self-preservation. For some, it involved renegotiating boundaries and, for others, it meant either supporting their partners in their recovery or disengaging from them completely.

The third theme '"It never ever goes away": the legacy of the attempt' underscores the extent to which the suicide attempt left a permanent imprint on almost every aspect of their lives. This imprint manifested psychologically, emotionally, and, for some, physically. The event reactivated childhood traumas for some participants and for others, it exacerbated underlying physical conditions. Hypervigilance also lay just beneath the surface and became the reason why participants avoided getting too comfortable with partners or children in case suicide were to revisit them. Some participants also experienced significant growth as a consequence of the experience: they described emerging from it with an enhanced outlook on life, enhanced personal strength, and enhanced relationships.

You are about to be abruptly introduced to all five interview participants in the chapters that follow. Abrupt in the sense that it mirrors, to a degree, their own experience of being abruptly and unceremoniously exposed to the suicide attempt of the person they considered themselves to be closest to in the world. They comprise one man and four women – 'Evan', 'Alice', 'Margaret', 'Carla' and 'Tanya'. I have given them pseudonyms in order to protect their anonymity. Their personal accounts are written in a manner that weave back and forth among them in order to reflect moments of convergence and divergence.

CHAPTER 2

Suffering the trauma of the attempt:
'It put nearly ten years on my life'

Participants were majorly impacted by the traumatic force of their partner's attempts. Their ability to recall minute details of the incident during the interview and the ease and speed with which they could tap back into the feelings they had during this time reflected the extent to which this experience had been permanently embedded within their psyche. Everything they knew or *thought* they knew about the world, themselves and their relationships was at once thrown into disarray which made for a tumultuous and inevitably life-changing event. Participants were exposed to so much in one fell swoop that they experienced a traumatic assault on their senses. The experience brought them spiritually closer to death because they had now faced their partners' attempted suicides. Furthermore, their perception that the trauma had substantially aged them brought them mentally closer to their own deaths.

Set against the backdrop of intense stress that they initially experienced, participants launched into action in a frantic attempt to save their partners' lives. They experienced their shock in waves, as if they were being 'hit' and scarred by the enormity of what had happened over the weeks and months that followed. Despite having just been 'through the wars', participants still had to honour obligations to work and family as well as come to terms with what their partners had done. They instantly felt overwhelmed by their need to put the pieces of the puzzle together and bombarded themselves with questions that needed answers as soon as humanly possible.

'It's a shock that comes in waves'

Utter terror, uncertainty and raw pain repeatedly crashed down on both participants and partners after the discovery of the suicide attempts and during the events that ensued. They were forced to confront the near ending of significant relationships through potential deaths that would have been both violent and self-inflicted. Four participants found their partners hanged or overdosed while one participant endured the arduous task of waiting for her husband to be found. In each case, none of the participants knew if their partners were dead or alive. No participant had prior exposure to a suicide attempt of a significant other, which made this experience personally uncharted territory. In the days and months following the attempt, participants continued to experience intrusive images, shock, and anxiety at a depth that was exceptionally unsettling for them. This challenged their assumptions about the world, which they had come to take for granted.

You will notice in the pages that follow that many of the extracts from the interviews and my analyses of them are written in the present tense. This makes the experience all the more 'live' for the reader and helps us to get a palpable sense of the event for all concerned.

Evan's wife had a history of anxiety and depression and had received psychiatric care, both as an in-patient and a day-patient, for a number of years at the time of her suicide attempt. Evan, similar to the other participants, experienced the time leading up to his partner's suicide attempt as unremarkable in that nothing in particular stood out to him looking back. In fact, on the night of her attempt, they had been entertaining friends, which he assumed they both had enjoyed. Later that night, however, his high spirits come to an abrupt and violent halt when he gets out of bed and finds his wife overdosed in another part of their home. His conceptualization of it as a 'show-stopper' reflects the depth of his shock:

> It's huge ... it's a show-stopper in your world ... I mean, you're faced with the finality of life or ... you don't know whether ... you're bringing somebody in [to hospital] that's about to die or are you bringing somebody in that can be brought back or ... it's a complete and utter show-stopper for you.

When he finds his wife's body, it brings into sharp focus his belief that the world as he knows it has transformed forever and so, too, he is transformed. Evan finds it intensely stressful and anxiety-provoking to not fully comprehend that with which he is faced. Is he rescuing a spouse who is very close to death but still has a chance of life or is he essentially recovering a body? His train of thought is now bombarded with uncertainty about his wife's future, his future, and their future together. Evan's shock is like an agonizing pain that comes and goes as he battles to transport his wife to A&E by car. He is exasperated by his obligation to provide mundane details to staff such as her name, date of birth, and condition. He is ultimately left alone with her in a cubicle, a situation that subsequently deteriorates into mayhem:

> She was all clammy an' all, but after about fifteen minutes ... I noticed her colour had completely changed, she had completely stopped breathing, so I lay her back on the table and ran around getting people ... so the emergency team came up and they jumped on her, and started trying to resuscitate her, eventually they had to put the panels on her chest ... and bring her back and it was a result of leaving her with me and what happened was, she had actually choked on her own vomit as a result of the stuff they had given her which was quite incredible.

Evan witnesses this incredible event knowing that only a short time ago he and his wife, who is now lying stripped and lifeless on a hospital trolley, had been entertaining friends in their garden.

He described himself as someone who ordinarily has a poor memory but, due to the enormity of this event, he is certain that it will be etched in his memory forever and that it has transformed him:

But I can recall the doctor straddling [wife's name], I can recall the doctor's face, I can recall the words she used, I can recall the people around, I can bring myself into that moment in a heartbeat ... where there's a little bubble of light, I'm here, I know who's standing here, here and there, that's how vivid an impression that made on my life, on my memory, and again I have a bad memory, so ...

Alice and her husband lead busy, professional lives and his job requires absences from home for several days at a time. They were in many respects like 'ships passing in the night' and communicated for the most part about practical issues and their children with little time set aside for each other. When Alice finds his lifeless body, her entire world comes crashing down in an instant around her and she is shocked into paralysis:

And I went down to the shed and I opened the door and there he was with the rope around one of the joists and around his neck. So, I froze, I stood there, I froze. And I looked and I says, 'Are you joking me?' and I'll never forget the look in his eyes. They were ... dead, his eyes were dead in his head. He just didn't care.

Due to her levels of utter shock, disbelief, and fear, she struggles to process what her senses are telling her, so much so that she initially thinks it can only be some kind of malicious joke. She recalls that the memory of his eyes haunted her. To her, they communicated that he had not only given up on life but also on her and their relationship.

Alice continues to be hit intermittently by shock in the hours following the attempt as she fights for his survival. Her world, as she knows it, has become unrecognizable to her. She finds herself in the extraordinary position of driving her husband to a psychiatric hospital but feels as though the man in the seat next to her has been possessed by a sinister force. While she is overcome with emotion and taking in every ounce of him, he appears numb to emotion and numb to her. Alice feels completely isolated in that whatever she is feeling seems irrelevant to him:

> *He never spoke, never opened his mouth, he had a cigarette, that was it. Even the colour of his face was just like grey ... it's as if, as if somebody had drained all the blood out of him. There was no emotion ... his eyes were something that you would see as if he were possessed. They were just focused on, in front of him, never looked sideways nothing just straight in front of him, never looked at me.*

She is dumbfounded when she is informed by hospital staff that there is nothing they can do for her husband and so, the onus, she feels, is on her to manage this situation. In this moment, she feels very much alone with this major responsibility and, for this reason, she needs to keep her shock in check to manage the situation. She believes that she would have at least *some* idea about how to proceed in other critical incidents but to cope with an actively suicidal spouse is something for which she is utterly ill-equipped in every sense:

> *I felt as if I was on my own. This was ... this never happened to me before, like, God, if somebody was after having a child you'd know what to do, if somebody was after having an accident you'd know what to do. But this was completely ... beyond. I couldn't believe what they were asking me to do. I really and truly, even to this day, I can't believe what they asked me to do and expected me to do.*

Margaret described a marriage that had been challenging for a long time as her husband suffered from depression and had problematic drinking habits. On the afternoon of his suicide attempt, he locked Margaret out of their home while she was out and took an overdose of antidepressant medication. Although he appeared to have simply fallen asleep, Margaret could none the less intuitively perceive the extraordinary in this relatively benign scene. She knew that a crisis was unfolding before her and that her life would never be the same again.

She describes, like some other participants, the sense that she is less in touch with reality, as if she is playing some kind of 'role' to manage the shock. For her, the experience is like she is set to automatic pilot or controlled by another in some way:

> *It's not logic, you just work on impulse ... some other part takes over and you do things ... as if you're governed*

by somebody else maybe ... you do whatever you think and I knew I couldn't open the door, so I just had to get somebody else to open the door, so then we called the ambulance, I think at that stage, and he was brought to hospital.

Margaret is, in effect, engaging parts of herself, both cognitively and behaviourally, that she doesn't recognize while simultaneously attempting to counteract the intensity of feeling so overwhelmed and out of control. She thinks that she is not engaging logic, but it transpires that she is incredibly focused and logical. Margaret felt that she had been emotionally in 'freeze' mode, that is, she had been prioritizing 'doing' over 'feeling'. As she recounts the experience, she moves back and forth between past and present tenses, which demonstrates how it is never fully in the past for her:

At the time, you wouldn't be feeling, you would just be doing. Like you don't feel, I don't ... you're not angry or anything, you just feel you must do whatever ... At the time, it was ... a bit numb ... it's like ... you just wait. I think you're in the lap of the Gods or sort of depending on others.

Tanya's husband failed to come home on the night of his suicide attempt. As he is a man you could ordinarily set your watch by, she instinctively knows that something isn't right. Her shock is akin to living through something in the realm of the 'real' while simultaneously experiencing it as 'surreal' and catastrophic in its impact. It is going against the usual order of things in her life and she grapples with the notion that people are not where they are *supposed* to be. Her husband is missing, and her family and friends have stepped outside of their own lives to support her through this terrifying experience:

> *This is Tuesday morning, everyone's supposed to be at work ... the world is supposed to be normal, I wasn't supposed to have woken up to this, this morning ...*

Tanya's world continues to disintegrate around her when her husband is finally located and it is confirmed that he has overdosed. It is only in A&E that her emotions finally catch up with her and she oscillates between shock and exhaustion. She appears to be struggling to figure out a procedure where there is none. Should she prioritize understanding how all of this came about or resign herself to comforting her dying husband?

> *You're going through these surges of adrenaline, like nearly to palpitations and sweat level to just, 'Oh please let me just lie down on the floor and sleep' through 'Would you, for God's sake, quickly tell me what happened before you die in case you're dying because I still don't know if you're dying' to 'Oh, dear God, if you're dying well then let's just hold hands for your last few hours and I'm not going to disturb your last', you know, 'if you've done what you've done' ...*

Many participants described the experience as all the more stressful and lonely because they couldn't turn to their partners for support. They had to manoeuvre their way through these life-changing events on their own while struggling to see an end in sight:

> *I presume it's up there with bereavement and divorce and moving house, it has to be up there as one of the most stressful situations, certainly it was the most stressful thing that has ever happened to me because – and I mean I've been through situations, my mother had been ill and took a while to die and it was awful ... but never been through anything like this and it went on and on and on because it was like ... if the person you love has an accident there's rehabilitation and there's an end point, that could be all physically and emotionally draining but now you find out the person you love chose to die with their own hand and leave you and your [daughter] because of a perceived situation, a historical situation that could have been – something could have been done about, it's a shock that comes in waves.*

As with Alice, Tanya feels that if he had had an accident of some kind there would be an established intervention, namely, rehabilitation that would encompass a prognosis and a care plan. Her husband's suicide attempt, however, has left her completely at sea regarding what the future holds for her. Here Tanya is suggesting that she doesn't see an end point for her regarding her partner's suicide attempt. The 'shock that comes in waves' represents the recurrent impact this has on her. Tanya uses the term 'the person you love' twice which perhaps reinforces the depth of pain she is experiencing. From her perspective, she sees his attempt as a 'decision' to leave her and she believes his actions were ultimately unwarranted. This provides some insight into her bubbling resentment towards him for the traumatic impact it has had on her life.

Carla's marriage had been slowly disintegrating for several years and she felt that the cracks were particularly apparent just prior to her husband's suicide attempt. Her husband's mental health had been deteriorating for a year and a half. He attended a psychiatric hospital as an in-patient for a period of six weeks. He and Carla had agreed to enter into couple counselling after this time. Two days after he is discharged from hospital, she is shocked to find her husband overdosed. In stark contrast to her expectations that they would engage in couple counselling so that she could reconnect with her husband, she is faced with the prospect of widowhood. Her experience is so traumatic that she has gaps in her memory:

> It was our son's birthday and my children were in the house ... and the babysitter was in one room and the children were in another room and he was in the room in the middle when I found him. I have no idea how or what happened for my child's birthday. I know someone took over that day and attended ... because I was obviously in the hospital and meeting with his family. In addition, when he woke up, I think he was actually given the last rites ...

The juxtaposition of the ordinary with the *extraordinary* is something that Carla finds almost impossible to process. These contrasts include the innocence of sleeping children in one room versus the stillness of their father overdosed in the adjoining room and the impending celebration of a child's birthday juxtaposed with his father receiving the last rites.

Carla acknowledges the epic proportions of this event but she is all too aware that if she faces the *extent* of her shock, it will send her 'over the edge' and cause further casualties, including both herself and her children:

> ... *My life had just crashed in the sense of something monumental had just happened in my life. There was no sense of 'happy days, out of here, it's done'. There was nothing like that, because there was so much stuff around it and, obviously, his own family, the way they were around it and we had two children in the middle of it all. Where was I for them? I was capable of being there, I'd say ... being there holding myself together was about as much as I could do.*

Carla describes a process of 'holding' herself together, which perhaps suggests that she imagined that she would have to brace herself against the next wave of shock to avoid falling apart altogether. She may also have experienced feelings of guilt related to her perception that she could have done more to protect her children at the time.

The walking wounded

Following their partners' suicide attempts, participants were faced with the double-edged process of continuing to meet life's practical obligations while also dealing with the extreme emotional fallout in the days, weeks and months afterwards. While their partners had given up on life and attempted to escape it, they found no escape from their immediate responsibilities: employment, care of children, financial obligations, roles within their community, obligations to friends and wider family, and of course, continuing to relate in *some* capacity to their spouse. What might have been viewed only yesterday as a mundane, routine task, today became a debilitating chore as they were effectively a 'man' down due to their partners' incapacitation.

As they tried to keep their heads above water financially and in other ways, participants struggled to digest what their partners had done and to negotiate a new dynamic within their relationships beyond the suicide attempts. They had to come to terms with the fact that their partners had *chosen* not to share their pain with them during a critical time in their lives. This caused them to re-evaluate how they conceptualized the relationship in a past, present, and future context. Participants struggled with a barrage of emotions about this, including loss, fear, rejection, anger, betrayal, regret, and responsibility, which most of them kept hidden for fear that they would be ridiculed socially. Although *their* worlds had crashed, the world kept turning regardless and, so, participants *had* to move forward while tending to these open wounds.

Alice felt the pressure of trying to keep everyone's heads above water following her husband's suicide attempt. As her husband falls into a zombie-like state, she effectively becomes a single mother fighting to pick up the pieces of their shattered family life:

> I had to worry about him, I had to worry about a mortgage to be paid. I had to worry about kids needing stuff for school. There was no income coming, well … my part-time income had to be put on hold 'cause I couldn't go to work. There was nobody I could even go out there and say, 'Well can you help with the mortgage, can you help me with this?'. Didn't want to know, didn't want to know.

Alice repeatedly mentions her worry here which conveys both the pressure to maintain some semblance of normality for her children and the overwhelming fear of losing what she has in her life, namely, her husband, her home, and the life they have built together. Even though he is functioning in a zombie-like state, Alice is unsure whether he still harbours the desire or has the capacity to attempt to take his life for a second time. As a result, she feels constantly on edge and finds herself 'looking over her shoulder' to prevent a possible recurrence of this while on *her* 'watch':

> I had no trust … because if he could do it once and he was in such a dark place … if there's tablets left there, Lexapro, like that's like handing a gun to a fella who's gonna go

out on a shooting spree ... so any sort of medication in the house had to be hidden. But that wasn't because of him, that was because of me. This was where the 'psycho' comes into it ... I was frightened to even leave a cough bottle in the house. I was frightened to leave anything that, in case he wanted to make another attempt and succeed the next time ... that he wasn't going to do it on my watch basically and I know that might sound selfish or whatever but I always had a fear of going out to work, the two kids away at school and I'd be at work and I'd come home and I'd find him.

Alice describes herself here as a 'psycho', which refers to the torment she experienced in her efforts to micro-manage every aspect of her husband's life so that history would not repeat itself. Although he attempted to hang himself, all Alice can see around her are further means of suicide whether it is anti-depressants or cough mixture. She mentions her fear of facilitating another suicide attempt but describes handing a 'gun' over to someone who shoots others rather than shooting themselves. This may provide insight into Alice's belief that, as with his past suicide attempt, a further attempt would inflict harm on her and her children rather than solely on him.

She juggles her immediate concerns for her husband's safety with her profound sense of loss for the closeness and shared outlook on life she had perceived them to have. When she compares the countless occasions when he communicated with her about issues that didn't really matter to all the opportunities he had to confide in her about things that *actually* caused him concern, a sense of utter betrayal comes strongly to the fore for her:

> *The hatred I had towards him was because ... everything we both worked for and our dreams and everything ... we could talk about everything and anything, and why all of a sudden was I blocked out and he couldn't talk to anybody. I hated, I felt as if that ... he betrayed me ... oh it's OK to talk to me if ... the tyre blew up in the lorry or his clothes weren't washed properly, or dinner wasn't nice or ... but yet you couldn't talk to me when there was something that* really *mattered in your head. And I felt that he didn't trust me to talk to me.*

Alice experiences a roller-coaster of emotions here due to her perception that his suicide attempt has nullified or, at least, threatened the very fabric of their relationship and all they shared. Her use of the term 'blocked' perhaps evokes an image of her partner slamming a door in her face or erecting barricades to keep her on the outside. For her, this provokes an issue about whether they can fundamentally trust each other.

Tanya's level of devastation was palpable. She felt deeply wounded that she had been kept completely in the dark regarding her husband's turmoil. Tanya felt that he had rejected not only her but also their daughter. Her maternal instincts came to the surface as she fought to protect her from the reality of the situation and its aftermath. Therefore, her first and *only* priority became the welfare of her daughter:

She was now living in a very confusing world where her
father had been whisked away, gone to one hospital,
gone to another hospital, came home – she had a father
that had basically come to ignore her or had very little to
do with her and me 24/7, to having both of us 24/7, so it
was a very stressful few months within the house. You're
conscious of your relationship, my relationship with her,
watching out for her.

In addition to the pressures to respond on a practical
level to their partners' suicide attempts, participants
simultaneously experienced a profound sense of loss. For
some, their loss related to their confrontation of the unhealthy
dynamic that had existed for much of their married life. For
others, the loss came with the realization that their partners
had turned away from them in their darkest hour rather
than towards them. This challenged their assumptions about
the states of their marriages and, indeed, about the identities
of the people with whom they fell in love.

Tanya shares Alice's sentiment in that she views her
husband's actions as the 'ultimate betrayal' of their relationship.
She views it as the 'ultimate' treachery because, to her, there
is little else that could surpass it now that he has broken her
trust, excluded her, deceived her, and turned away from her at
the most critical time in their lives:

I lived with a person that I thought I knew inside out,
I thought we had great friendship, you're soulmates,
we were good together and I found out then that the

person I lived with and loved did not turn to me during his – what you would call the greatest crisis in his life and I remember trying to tell people at the time, to varying reactions, that I saw this as a complete and utter ultimate betrayal of our relationship which I put on a par with – I said to friends your husband, you know, runs off with another woman, runs off with another man, runs off, gambles the house from under you, various scenarios, or commits suicide, like, where would you put it? And different people, obviously in the heightened emotion of the situation, had different reactions but I would pretty much have put suicide – I would have put suicide up there quite highly.

Evan's outlook on his wife's suicide attempt was quite different to other participants because, for years before this, he had taken a very active role in helping her to get the best support possible to improve her mental health. However, her attempt is completely unexpected and leaves him dazed and deeply upset. Despite his sadness, he needs to find a way to move forward and does so by 'aggressively' advocating for her through the mental health system to find a 'solution':

... what becomes very clear is that if you don't have somebody batting for you, putting you centre of ... if you can't do it yourself ... of your own mental health, or your own health, whether it be mental or physical, in the system, you just become part of it, you won't be getting the actual treatment you need ... so you do absolutely

need somebody that's willing to look out for you, willing to shout for you, willing to talk for you ... if you can't do it for yourself.

The metaphor 'batting' suggests that, regardless of what he is experiencing as a result of her attempt, he must fight for her in some way or it will be his fault that she becomes a *part* of the system. Since his wife is not in a fit state to 'bat' for herself, Evan feels the pressure to maintain his stamina to prevent the situation from deteriorating further.

For Evan, his wife's suicide attempt reignites a sense of loss that he experienced a number of years earlier when she entered a psychiatric hospital for the first time. He knows intuitively that her suicide attempt is another defining moment that will inevitably change how he sees her and the relationship forever:

... but I remember walking out of there and I remember saying to myself ... 'OK, the person I loved and married has gone because the person that's going to come out of there, no matter what, or how you look at it, no matter how you dress it up, because of the very nature of what they're going through, is going to be adversely changed.' So you're sort of thinking to yourself ... 'OK, so who's going to come in, will it be someone I like less, will it be someone I like more, will it be someone I can deal with more, will it be someone I can deal with less?' ... it's all that coming.

Evan is suggesting here that her suicide attempt could herald a fundamental change in who she is. He describes his anticipation about who she will become. He believes that the person with whom he fell in love is gone and that, while the stranger in her place will look like his wife, she may think, feel, and behave in ways that he will not be able to love.

A desperate search for answers

All participants were exposed to an event of extraordinary proportions that was far removed from the 'everydayness' of their lives. Without a tangible framework within which to process the experience, participants engaged in a frantic and fraught attempt to develop plans of action and to understand their partners' motivations to attempt suicide. For some, the period of time during which their partners' whereabouts were unknown was fraught with just as many unanswered questions as they had when they located them and learned of their suicide attempts. Their search for answers to a throng of questions was a desperate act in that, the sooner they gained insight, the easier it would be to begin the task of putting their lives back together. It also answered the very human call to gain relief from ambiguity and allowed participants to regain a sense of control in an otherwise out-of-control experience.

Alice recalled her burning desire to know exactly why her husband tried to kill himself. She believes that if she can understand what he was going through emotionally at the time of the attempt, piece by piece, it will aid in her *own* processing of the experience. Alice is incredibly frustrated, however, by the painfully slow way her husband is communicating *anything* to her:

I was so fed up tryin' to … pull the words from his mouth for him to talk, for him to try and tell me was there a reason, if there was a reason, could he talk about it? For me to get my head around it, I wanted answers from him.

Her lack of answers creates a significant blind spot for Alice, which in turn creates both significant worry for her husband and anger towards him. Without the complete picture, Alice is unsure if he will repeat the act:

It was just the complete worry, the annoyance, the fear. Like the fear of not knowing I think makes you angry too.

Alice moves relentlessly back and forth along a continuum from an almost obsessive desire to gain *any* kind of information from him, to toying with her own ideas about what happened, to believing that the answers she seeks don't actually exist:

So something went, something triggered, something happened and I don't think he can explain it because he doesn't know himself. And that's why I think people like myself and other people, 'til the day we die we're always gonna say 'but why?' And I don't think there is any answers for it.

All of the participants had very individual styles of communication with their partners and, consequently, some looked directly to their partners for explanations while others looked outside of their relationship for answers.

Margaret recalled that virtually nothing was said between her and her husband about his suicide attempt because she believed that he would deny it was intentional. She doesn't force the issue as she is unsure whether she could face any explanation from him. She also creates distance between herself and the experience by depersonalizing it; she imagines how a person *in general* could make sense of it rather than her in particular. Like Alice, Margaret moves backwards and forwards between the belief that there are no answers to why he attempted suicide and the sense that she intuitively knows that some kind of rationale for his attempt exists:

> *There is no sense. There is no actual black and white ... for anyone who does suicide, I don't think there's an explanation. There's certainly not an easy one.*

In the absence of answers, Margaret turns to hospital staff to give her any semblance of understanding. The extent of her husband's alcoholism is highlighted and consequently becomes one explanation for his suicide attempt:

> *He was in hospital and then he was in [name of psychiatric hospital] in [location] for a couple of weeks after that and he was being treated for alcohol addiction ... and they told me at the time that he was never going to ... stop ... that he didn't have a pattern of stopping and that was their opinion and so I had*

to decide whether I could live with that or not and I decided to live with it rather than walk ... that I could live with somebody who ... as long as I knew that he probably wasn't going to stop drinking ... you always hope somebody will change.

Margaret now has to face up to the news that her husband's alcoholism is unlikely to be a temporary phenomenon and, consequently, she must let go of her former hope that he would eventually stop. She is now faced with another critical question to answer: Is she prepared to battle on in the relationship or should she say goodbye to it?

Evan's wife had been involved with mental health services for a number of years before her suicide attempt due to anxiety and panic attacks. Her suicide attempt was unexpected but *unsurprising* to him because they had been on a merry-go-round within the public health system and had felt as if they were getting nowhere. As an advocate for her, he had been trying to get answers about how best to deal with her illness for years, but he had felt ignored. It was only after her attempt that he realized that the 'answer' did not reside in any previous intervention they had received, whether in-patient treatment, day-patient care, or the array of psychotropic medication she had been prescribed:

I think I felt empowered again in the sense that I was able to say ... 'OK' ... you know, it's not just my perception. I've been thinking this for a long time now, but it's actual, now I don't have to, now it's actual that the system's not working, it doesn't work, so everything we've done up to this point, you can wrap it up and fuck it away.

Evan's renewed energy is possibly sourced from a multitude of emotions including anger and the resentment he feels towards those who did not listen to him. He now uses it to find the *right* answer so that his wife can begin to show signs of recovery. 'Wrapping it up and fucking it away' denotes Evan's frustration and anger towards the professionals who have let him down or, perhaps more significantly, towards himself for not acting sooner on his hunch that the system was not working for her. Evan describes 'waking up' to the inefficacy of the interventions so far. It is bittersweet in that he is finally able to let go of the expectations he had, but this immediately creates an urgency to find an alternative answer to prevent a possible second attempt that could succeed:

I know now absolutely what's been happening to date is not working, so now I have the freedom myself to let that go. The awakening in the sense of this ... OK, there has to be something else, there has to be a different way, no concept or notion of what that was, where it was going to be, where I was going to find it or whatever ... it was no more than that. It was just an awakening that ... if we continue on the way we're going to go, we're going to end up quite possibly around a grave ...

Tanya was bombarded with a barrage of questions both internally and from friends and family who rallied together to locate her husband during the hours he was missing. After she becomes worried about her husband's well-being, she quickly finds herself immersed in impossible questions about the appropriateness of her response and its implications:

> *I didn't know at what stage to do what, I mean do you start contacting people and then it turned out he's fallen asleep somewhere, you know that, do you make a fool of yourself versus how quickly do you act?*

Tanya is conscious of how people in her life will evaluate her. This bears out later when she reflects on what assumptions others will make about why he tried to end his life. She was certain that one of two things had happened: either he had had a 'breakdown' and he was missing somewhere or he had killed himself. In her desperation, Tanya tries to imagine walking in his shoes during this crisis in an attempt to establish his whereabouts, but this exercise fails miserably:

> *Where are you? If you had spent 28 years with somebody, married 24 at that stage, with him 28, so been with him more of my life than I wasn't with him ... if two souls are entwined in such close – soulmates, should I not know in my guts or heart and soul, whatever, where he was? That's just the – thinking on that level. Should I not know?*

Tanya embroils herself in self-doubt and criticizes herself for not having an intuitive knowledge about her partner's inner world given that he is a man she has known for almost three decades. She feels weighed down by the expectation of both herself and others that she will come up with answers and resolve this ordeal for everyone concerned. Subsequent to locating her husband, Tanya's desperate search for answers intensifies. She shifts her focus to confirming whether he has attempted suicide and, if so, identifying his motives. The strength of her desire to understand 'why?' almost surpasses her compassion towards him during the period when she is unsure if he is going to survive. Dissatisfied with the mumbled utterances from him in his hospital bed, Tanya's patience is tested as she battles conflicting feelings of pity, frustration, and resentment:

> *I then do start, I think, needing a bit more: 'Why …
> What has happened? Why?' … So you start the why,
> when, what, where sort of – nothing makes sense
> … there's phrases, half-phrases, half-sentences … it's
> exhaustion on his part and inability to articulate and
> he's looking at me as if to say, 'I've already told you this'
> and I'm going, 'You haven't', a growing resentment that
> he knows why he did it, I think his sister knows why he
> did it, his brother obviously knows why he did it, I think
> I need to know why he did it.*

CHAPTER 3

Adjusting in the wake of the attempt
'It shifted the whole world on its axis'

Participants went through the difficult process of adjustment in order to withstand the 'seismic' shift that the whole experience entailed. This was a very active experience for participants. They ebbed and flowed in their thinking and behaviour to make sense of how this could have happened and to work out how best to remain functioning. They were forced to wrestle with some dark feelings about both themselves and their partners. An unavoidable part of this journey involved thrashing out whom or what was responsible for their partners trying to kill themselves.

It was an uncomfortable but necessary process to go through in order to move forward. Participants were tormented by negative thoughts about their ability to cope with the situation and about the status and quality of their relationships. In an attempt to withstand this torment, participants developed various means of self-preservation. For some, it involved renegotiating boundaries and, for others, it meant supporting their partners in their recovery or disengaging from them completely. The adjustment endured by participants in the wake of the attempt transformed their view of themselves, their partners, and their outlooks on life.

The blame game

'The blame game' denotes participants' back-and-forth 'finger-pointing' about *whom* or *what* 'drove' their partners to attempt to take their own lives. This was a natural progression in their desperate search for answers. They experienced conflicting thoughts and feelings about how they found themselves in these circumstances; for some participants, it was more clear-cut than for others. The source of their conflict was internal, external, or a combination of the two. It could be internal in the sense that they perceived that they were in some way directly responsible for 'driving' their partners to suicide. This was more often to do with something they had *not* done for their partners; therefore, they experienced guilt by omission.

It could be external in the sense that participants blamed circumstances that were largely beyond their control. For some, however, they felt that responsibility ultimately lay with the individual who attempted to take their own life. While unpleasant, playing the 'the blame game' was a necessary evil to make any sense of the experience. The attempt to discover culpability at least helped partners to put the puzzle pieces together and, ultimately, it facilitated the adjustment process.

In the wake of her husband's attempt, Alice is adamant that she has failed him as a wife and best friend. She is plagued with intrusive thoughts about what she *could* have done differently to prevent this, especially because she believed they were best friends:

> *But it was coming on him and I think everything just came to a head then, and really and truly the way I felt was I felt guilty I didn't see it happening, I didn't see it coming, I didn't see the tell-tale signs, I seen nothing, absolutely nothing, and so I was angry with myself then ... because this was my best friend ...*

She believes that there were definite precursors to his attempt one of which was depression, which she perceived as an illness that *came upon* him like an outside force. She chastises herself for failing to see it coming and for failing to act upon it sooner. Alice also holds society and its support systems accountable for his suicide attempt as they both have failed in her eyes to champion mental health, in particular, that of men. Had society encouraged men to be more emotionally demonstrative rather than thrusting a 'big boys don't cry' attitude on them and had hospitals made a more concerted effort to highlight the warning signs, she believes her husband would never have found himself in this situation:

> *... there's no signs out there, nobody gives information about this, nobody says if a man's depressed they shouldn't cry, they're tellin' ya not to cry. It's the way they grew up basically, that you know, you're a big hard man, you're a big tough nut, you'll be fine, and they're not, they're really not ...*

Tanya recounts a stark transition from the hyperactivity of the search for her husband to waiting in Accident and Emergency. Only when the dust begins to settle does she have the 'headspace' to begin thinking about what motivated his behaviour. As with Alice, her automatic conclusion is that she is guilty of a crime and that others will uphold this verdict since, in her mind, she has somehow *driven* him to suicide:

Well ... when a wife's murdered, the first suspect is the husband ... when someone commits suicide and dies, 'Well I don't think they were too happy anyway' ... had [husband's name] succeeded I'm the first suspect, I'm the one that would have had to wear the T-shirt that said, 'Actually, it wasn't my fault', do you know what I mean? He said, 'This is nothing to do with you.' Of course I'm the first suspect ... I'm saying suspect – I would be the one that would ... [ask] someone else, who drives somebody to suicide? Their partner!

Tanya is wary of how others will perceive her and likens herself to a prime suspect in a murder inquiry. She seems convinced that others will point the finger at her and consequently she feels obliged to try to 'clear' her name.

Participants were forced to grapple with the near deaths of their life partners, which went against the natural order of things. They had assumed that they would both pass away in their old age, but they were forced to look the finality of life square in the eye instead due to their partners' attempts. For some participants, knowing that this was the case was just too difficult to ignore and they blamed their partners for these traumatic events. The more information Tanya received about her husband's behaviour leading up to his attempt, the more she felt that the blame should lie with him. She learned that his attempt was well thought out and that he had planned it months in advance of the act:

> *You have been planning to do this and what? Sat opposite me eating dinner, like? You! And you can go on and extrapolate that on to all the normal mundane things which weave together a family life, a relationship, a – you don't think on the bigger level, I actually thought, I actually thought of the smaller, more mundane: you looked into my eyes at one stage,* knowing *you were going to kill yourself,* so what – looking into my eyes not good enough to stop you? So, why wasn't I enough to stop you? Why was our daughter not enough to stop you? Why – so yeah, there is an actual part now of resentment, annoyance, there wasn't anger because you couldn't have but feel ultimately so sorry for this person, this man you loved lying in a hospital bed, you know what I mean?

Tanya powerfully describes the raw hurt and pain she feels now that she knows that he interacted with both her and their daughter on a daily basis, looked into their eyes and chatted about the mundane; yet all the while he had a plan in place. She was perplexed that neither she nor her daughter seemed worthy 'enough' for him to reconsider suicide. Tanya ultimately found his actions wanting and selfish in the extreme.

Margaret also feels the weight of responsibility for her husband. This was imposed on her by in-laws *before* his suicide attempt, which probably added to her sense of responsibility and guilt after his attempt. This only increases her confusion about the part she has played in all of this. Despite the culture at the time that shunned open communication, she firmly believes that her particularly poor communication skills promoted his suicidal behaviour:

> *Could I have done more? Could I have ... talking would have been one of them, not necessarily ... it's one of the hardest, I think, to sort of sit down and have a ... I would still find it the hardest. I can talk all day but not, you know ... it's ... again, it's running away from the hard bits, not ignoring them.*

Following interactions with psychiatric personnel, however, Margaret simultaneously holds an opposing belief that she could *never* hold the power to either cause suicidal behaviour in another person or, indeed, keep them from harm's way:

> *Yeah, well, if somebody decided to do whatever, drive dangerously, drink and drive, it was ... I had no hand, act or part in it, you know what I mean. I didn't do it or could prevent it, that it was totally ... like I could only do what I thought was right in my life, I couldn't live somebody else's life for them, right or wrong.*

Margaret is perhaps alluding here to her husband's old habit of drink-driving and the sense of responsibility she had felt over the years because she had 'allowed' this reckless behaviour. She comes to the realization that he has *always* been in charge of his *own* actions whether drinking heavily, driving dangerously, or taking his own life.

For Carla, something clicks in her mind the moment she finds her husband overdosed. Even more strongly than Tanya, Carla lays the finger of blame squarely on her husband's shoulders. She absolves herself of the responsibility to 'mother' him. This is a defining moment for her in the sense that although she has taken on responsibility for his welfare in the past, this is an act that has crossed the line for her:

> *From when I found him, there was no doubt. I don't think I even attached to any negative feeling towards myself even having it ... I don't think I said, 'Oh, that's an awful thing' ... I don't think that came to me. I think it genuinely was so strong ... the feeling was so strong that I was crystal clear. I said, 'This relationship is over.' Not in an angry response to what he'd done, but in a ... as I said, crystal clear ... this is done, this is done.*

As was the experience of some other participants, Carla feels the finger of blame coming in her direction from in-laws who believe that she could have been more sympathetic towards him:

> *His parents and brothers and sisters who stepped in very*

quickly to have a meeting with me about what was going on and it was suggested that I hadn't shown enough TLC, you know, a bit more TLC would have made a big difference. That dimension was going on in the midst of it all.

Here Carla explains the extent to which her experience was multi-faceted. Her life as she knows it has just crashed; she desperately tries to process what has just happened. She must find a way to move forward. A further dimension is added to her turmoil when family members accuse her of lacking in 'tender loving care'. Carla, like most of the other participants, found that 'the blame game' negatively transformed her assumptions about herself, others, and the efficacy of the system.

Countering the 'torment': strategies for self-preservation

Participants were exposed to an experience of extraordinary proportions without any established language, behaviour, or response to guide them through it. Their backs were against the wall and, in stark contrast to their partners, they were going to do whatever it took to ensure self-preservation. They tapped into whatever resources were available; they threw caution to the wind at times and did or said things that might not have felt socially appropriate. All they could do was rely on life experience and instinct as much as possible to preserve their emotional, psychological, and physical well-being. Participants were strongly motivated to find antidotes to this torment and talked about the need to 'trust their own counsel' and 'take it on the chin' in an effort to avoid ending up in similar situations to their partners.

Shortly after his attempt, Alice has the sobering realization that her husband is not going to receive the kinds of support she had imagined there would be to deal with this crisis. As his next of kin, she feels that it falls to her to ensure he receives appropriate help. Neither immediate family nor in-laws have been told of his attempt. Her sons are not informed as she wants to protect them from the horror of what has happened and to protect their view of 'Dad' as their idol. As a result, Alice carries the load alone and talks several times about her desire to 'scream from the mountain tops' as a means of protecting her mental health. She knows that she needs to let go of this weight to preserve her own psychological and physical health:

> And I, I just said to him one day, I says look if that's what you want to do [kill himself] you go ahead and do it, I've done enough, I'm not stoppin' you, I can't stop you anymore, if that's the way you want to be, you go ahead and do it.

Her lack of knowledge about what help he needs coupled with the feeling that every door is being slammed in her face compels Alice to acknowledge that she has reached the 'end of her tether'. Alice's exasperation is evident as she abruptly tells him that it is not humanly possible for her to do any more. She hands the 'baton' to her husband to carry the responsibility for whether he lives or dies. Alice is encouraged by her husband's response to her ultimatum. When she is made aware that he is engaging well in counselling, this seems to make it easier for her to *re-engage* with him. Over time, she is more able to cope with what she perceives as a painfully slow process of recovery:

> *There was manys a night he cried in my arms and I just rubbed his hair or rubbed his shoulder, rubbed his back. He felt very insecure because he felt then that he was letting me down again. And, we had talks about it and I said, 'Look it, when things are right, we'll be fine, we are fine ... we have to get you better first ... when we get you better first, then we can work on other things.'*

Alice appears here to have found hope for her future again. This enables her to carry hope for both of them and to offer reassurance about the strength of their relationship during the times when her husband is particularly low. As her husband's well-being improves, they begin a journey of rediscovery and reacquaint themselves with one another. Alice highlighted that, for her, their effort to become friends again overcame her urge to 'shake' him at times. She mentioned frequently the extent to which the simple act of talking paid dividends to both of them and, ultimately, to their relationship:

> *So, we set boundaries for ourselves, we had a date night. We got to be friends again and that was the most important thing. And then on a Tuesday night was our date night. We got to know each other again*

... reminiscing on the past and when we were teenagers and anything to get his mind off that year and a half or so that he was in a very bad place.

The creation of boundaries encompassed a number of domains. These ranged from her call for her husband to take a more active role in household chores and with the children to their commitment to be more open and honest with one another about their feelings.

Throughout the interview, Evan gave the strong impression of a man relatively unperturbed by the trauma of his partner's suicide attempt with a strong focus on advocating for her and maintaining hope for her recovery. None the less, just beneath the surface, the attempt was having a huge drain on the relationship. He often had to 'dig deep' emotionally to stay the course:

One of the things that enabled me to stay was a little mantra I had with myself when things got really bad and that was ... 'get her better and then you can leave'. Now that's pretty powerful.

Evan was adamant that he had no intention of leaving her but took solace in knowing that the option existed. He described it as a 'little' mantra but later acknowledged how far-reaching the consequences would have been if he had followed through on it. His mantra reflected at the very least the duty of care he felt he had and, at most, the love he still felt for her. Evan talked at length about his motivation to get his wife better and very little about how he was coping. It appears, however, that he had a number of resources such as his mantra, which he implies was *one* of the things that enabled him to stay.

Evan knew that the only way his wife would ever turn a corner would be through her own motivation. He struggled, however, to see any evidence of this happening until she began proactively dealing with her anxiety. She joined a support group but, for the first four weeks or so, she sat in her car feeling too terrified to go in and join the other members. Evan could see past her non-attendance and saw evidence of progress instead and with that, came hope:

> *She'd come back ... 'How did you get on?' 'I didn't go in.' 'But you went', you know, but then to go the next week and do the same ... but there's a fire in there somewhere, isn't there? So there was no absolute conversations, but there was bits that you could see that were starting to make sense which was great, because I knew there had to be a complete change and I didn't know where it was going to come from and I suppose I least thought it was going to come from [wife's name], but it did.*

Evan talks here about the 'fire' for change that he could sense in his wife. This was a further resource for him, which kept him engaged in her recovery. He describes his belief that a sea change needed to occur, his pessimism about this happening, and his sense of reassurance when it did.

When the changes in his wife began to gather momentum,

this lightened the load considerably for Evan. The torment that had besieged him was countered with a sense of pride in his wife. He no longer viewed her as a helpless victim but as a master of her own destiny:

> *I see the suicide attempt as a metamorphosis, I absolutely see it as the caterpillar who thinks it's fucking dying and then turns into a butterfly.*

Evan provides powerful imagery here through his metaphor of the butterfly. It represents his wife's triumph over adversity and her transcendence following her self-imposed near-death experience. She had become something *more* than she was before the attempt.

What set Carla's experience apart from the other participants was her certainty that her life would deteriorate further were she to remain in the relationship. For her, her husband's attempt was the straw that broke the camel's back:

> *I had this image of me ... this very strong, visual image came to me of me in the corner fighting for my own life, that my survival depended on me leaving and that I chose to survive. That's where, I suppose, there was no turning back. I can't tell you that maybe we said we'd give it a go. I have no conscious memory of that. All I know is that, in that moment, I could see myself ... I can still see myself having this ... 'I'll die if I stay in this relationship'. I didn't mean physically, I meant emotionally I would have died inside. I was going to die inside.*

Carla emphasizes here her belief that her *own* life is in danger on the basis of this catastrophic event. She conceptualizes a life of emotional turmoil as a kind of death in itself. While her husband has conspired against life, she chooses to move towards it. Protecting her emotional life ultimately entails creating as much physical distance from her husband as possible.

Carla had to carry the weight of sole parenthood, keep her business going, and come to terms with leaving the marriage for both herself and her children. Her husband was effectively absent from their lives for the best part of three months around the time of his suicide attempt. One way in which she countered the torment was to be as cooperative as possible with him as the terms of the separation were agreed:

> We agreed on shared custody. I mean, we did all our legal work. Everything was done. There was no big fight, there was no throwing stones at each other, there was none of that. We did do it as ... that dreadful word ... 'amicably' as possible. How could you be anything else when you're in the throes of something like that? We did do it with as much grace as we could in the circumstances, both of us, I'd say.

Carla describes the term 'amicably' as 'dreadful', which perhaps implies that she was saddened by how cold and clinical the ending of their marriage was, devoid of the bond and emotion they once shared. None the less, she couldn't imagine experiencing it in any other way given what she was going through at the time.

Carla sang the praises of her good friends who were a tremendous support for her during her darkest moments when she felt devoid of energy and answers. Their positivity brought a welcome balance to her life at a time when she could have easily let the torment get the better of her:

I had a number of friendships that were incredibly supportive and I think they would have been a huge assistance in helping my self-esteem. I have a couple of relationships that would just have been so positive and yeah ... that would just have made such a difference to me... that would have been very supportive throughout the whole time.

Her self-worth was severely knocked in the wake of her husband's attempt on a number of fronts: she had been motivated to enter couple counselling with him just before his overdose, she felt accused by in-laws that she hadn't been adequately supportive of him, and she felt guilty that she was breaking up her children's home. The quality of her friendships acted as a buffer between her and the torment that ensued, and in due course, saw her come out the other end of it still intact.

CHAPTER 4

The legacy of the attempt
'It never ever goes away'

Participants experienced the trauma of their partner's suicide attempt as a permanent imprint on their psyches. This imprint manifested psychologically, emotionally, and physically. It brought vulnerabilities to the surface such as physical illness, repressed traumatic memories from childhood, and their transformed views of their relationships with their partners. All participants had a tumultuous time adjusting to the event and yet, paradoxically, all experienced personal growth including increased inner strength, enhanced relationships and more profound outlooks on life. These experiences inevitably transformed how they saw themselves, their partners, their worlds, and, indeed, their futures.

What lies beneath

Subsequent to their partner's suicide attempt, different forms of unseen or 'below surface' impact transpired for participants. The event reactivated childhood traumas and worsened underlying physical conditions. Hypervigilance also surfaced for participants in that they avoided getting too comfortable in case suicide were to revisit their partners or children. This became a hidden but ever-present feature of post-attempt life for some participants as their partners stood as constant reminders of the suicide attempts. They were also easily triggered by conversations or by media coverage of suicide or missing persons. The entire experience adversely transformed how participants saw their relationships with their partners.

Alice offered a rich insight into how her exposure to the stress of her husband's suicide attempt brought a mass of 'unfinished business' to the surface regarding her troubled childhood. She had felt supported over the years by her husband who was very familiar with her past:

> *He's always been there for me like all through my childhood and that and he knows about the abuse I went through and that and ... I'd be talking to him about it and talking to him about it and ... hand on heart [laughter] I don't know how he listened. I really don't know, I don't know how he stayed as sane for as long as he did. But that's what I'm saying like we know each other so well. But emm ... I think with him attempting this then it dug all this back up with me again.*

Not only did his attempt strike a familiar chord with her on a number of fronts but it also meant that her greatest champion was no longer available to support her. Her early story, which began with parental divorce and the loss of her childhood home, echoes many of the themes that she experienced on the basis of his attempt:

> So I haven't had much luck [laughter] with the HSE or doctors but ... that's what I'm on about with mental illness. My mother probably had a breakdown as well but she got very violent with it, she got very abusive, she got very ... an alcoholic like. And I'd have said to you before that I would've known about mental illness not from the husband but from somebody else. But ... she's a totally different person. Like ... she's just pure evil, really, really pure evil.

She describes a story of survival in which she needed to take extreme measures to keep things afloat, behaviour that bears a similarity to her response following his attempt. On reporting her own abuse, she felt the system was dismissive of her and, correspondingly, this was her experience in the aftermath of her husband's attempt.

While Alice also had previous exposure to mental illness through her mother, she differentiates between this experience and that of her husband. She viewed her husband as a victim of his breakdown whereas she suspected there to have been some degree of malevolence to her mother's breakdown. During my interview with Alice, she described the loss of her relationship with her father, a significant male figure in her life, which resonates with the near loss of her husband with whom she had a bond since childhood. When all of this surfaced at once, it came at a cost for Alice as it caused her to deteriorate both psychologically and emotionally.

While Evan feels thankful in many ways for the experience and is spiritually stronger as a result, Alice does not necessarily share this sentiment as she has had to adapt to a life in the shadow of her husband's suicide attempt:

> *You're actually frightened to get comfortable again in case there's another big upheaval. That's basically what it is ... I'm not saying you're living from day to day, that would be a lie. You're frightened to get too ecstatically happy, or plan too far ahead, or even to this day I would be the same ... I just take every day now as it comes.*

This powerful summation shows how differently she relates to the world in the wake of the attempt. Her daily life is now characterized by fear to varying degrees subject to her evaluation of how her husband is doing through his mood, tone of voice, facial expressions and so on. In essence, Alice has learned to live with the discomfort of knowing that the 'rug could be pulled from under her' at any point. Alice has created a new kind of template for how she relates to people she cares about, especially her children. This mode of behaviour comes from a place of real fear and carries with it the pressure to recognize 'tell-tale signs', signs she believes she should have seen in her husband:

> *Even with my two sons now ... they would be my life ... I can even see myself now [laughter] the ages they are, looking at them to see if there's any little tell-tale signs, if they're gettin' down in the dumps or if they're, anything*

like that or anything worrying them and they can talk to
me about anything and they know that.

Tanya was hurt and angered by the apparent lack of
consideration her husband demonstrated for both her and
their daughter through his attempt, especially because of his
knowledge of the early traumatic loss Tanya had experienced:

And he chose to leave her and shocking as it is that he
would choose to leave me, at least I was a grown adult
and I had chosen to marry and be with him, she did not
ask to be left without a father at ten years of age and I
think I became very angry, more on her behalf possibly,
maybe not, compounded by the fact that I lost my own
father at eight-and-a-half by – and through an accident
... and witnessed the Guards arriving at the door and he
knew how – that's an awful thing to happen to an eight-
and-a-half-year-old and I could picture a scenario that
had he succeeded, had he succeeded the Guards would
have arrived at my door ...

She was unsure whether her anger was more on behalf
of her daughter or herself. Since her daughter was similar in
age at the time of his suicide attempt to the age she was when
her own father was killed, it is likely that she began to have
a new appreciation for the confusion, pain, and anguish that
she experienced but couldn't understand as a child. Tanya
imagines what could have happened had her husband been
found dead and feels for her eight-year-old self.

Tanya's emotional fragility is paralleled with an ongoing physical condition that she is obliged to address despite the enormity of what has just occurred in her life. What should have been a fairly routine procedure and a straightforward recovery turns into a much more sinister and chronic condition:

> I'd had a medical procedure on my spine just the week before it which was bad timing on his part as well and it was another area of him not prioritizing. As a result of running around hospitals and sitting on plastic chairs outside consultants' rooms or whatever ... weeks later I collapsed ... and it had aggravated the procedure that I had had done on my back, over the months afterwards, it took – what should have been a pretty straightforward recovery, didn't recover, my health deteriorated ... afterwards I knew I wasn't getting any better but I didn't know if this was lapsed into the upset and confusion, if it was depression, it did turn out to be established medically ... I had an underlying condition which escalated and – into [a] much more chronic condition during the months after the suicide through which ... the medical personnel involved would no doubt [believe] that post-traumatic stress would be involved.

Tanya's ongoing anger and resentment towards her husband's actions are evident here. She views his actions as inconsiderate given what was happening in her life just before his attempt. She questions why her recovery was hampered to such an extent that she queries if she was suffering from depression. Perhaps, Tanya is sharing that she *did* in fact experience something akin to depression in the months following his suicide attempt. She is very certain, however, that she suffered symptoms of post-traumatic stress as a direct result of his suicide attempt. Confirmation by medical personnel of her post-traumatic stress diagnosis seems to be important to her, which may suggest that she felt it wouldn't have been taken seriously otherwise.

Tanya provides a powerful image of the trajectory that both she and her husband took at the point of his suicide attempt. For her, his attempt marked him having reached rock bottom and so, from then on, the only way was up for him. However, she felt that her emotional and physical health took a nosedive from the moment she knew he was missing:

The impact on him was that was his lowest point and he only got better after it because it all came out in the open, it was all established and he became stronger and better. The night of the suicide [attempt] was only the start of my downward journey and back up – does that make sense?

In her eyes, he was provided with everything he needed to make a solid recovery including therapy and regular contact with his family of origin. In the midst of her turmoil, however, Tanya felt pressure from in-laws to have him return as soon as possible to their marital home, which was something she didn't want. She also felt the weight of responsibility on her shoulders from psychologists to prevent a second suicide attempt. All of this was happening while her physical health deteriorated.

Of all the participants, Tanya's description of how her life changed after the attempt is the most saddening. The impact for her in terms of ongoing hurt and resentment is very tangible as she recounts a return to some form of 'normality':

So as things quietened down and people stopped asking, slowed down in asking, as he re-established his life and goes back to work and goes to football matches and goes to all these places, people stop asking and we should have returned to what people call normality. But I didn't get over it. And I don't think I ever will actually get over it.

What sets Tanya apart from the people in her life now is that, although they appear to be able to seamlessly slide back into the roles and day-to-day activities they pursued before the suicide attempt, her experience differs entirely. It is similar to how people describe life after they bury a loved one, when people stop calling or asking how things are. Her resentment towards her husband is very evident as she describes his re-engagement with life, whereas she feels that his suicide attempt is responsible for her disengagement from life. Tanya feels a social pressure to put it behind her, but she is not optimistic at all that she will be able to achieve this.

Something has changed in Tanya and, by association, something has changed in the relationship. She asserts that she will never again be able to one hundred per cent trust her husband. She eloquently describes how she experienced the relationship before the attempt and the devastating impact it has had on it since:

Our relationship was never the same again. Never. And I really don't think it ever will be because I know I'm not the same person I was, definitely I'm not the same person I was. I would rely on him less emotionally, I don't think he's my first sounding board, and I mean emotionally ... I think I'm actually probably stronger in some ways ... where I lived in the situation, what I perceived to be a massively open, loving relationship where he was both my best friend, the person I sounded, no – the person I turned to first about simple things like dinner ... right through to the big things in life. He's not my first point now because I think I would think more for myself first, work it through myself first and also I think – I think I don't respect or value his opinion as much.

Tanya emphasizes here that things have changed permanently and adversely so. Her reflex to share all those parts of her life that reflect closeness in a relationship has diminished entirely, from the everyday mundane to the most significant of life events. His suicide attempt has pushed her to trust her own judgement more but this is a bittersweet change as it has only come about through a loss of respect for her best friend.

Tanya talks about the suicide attempt in the past tense but it is very evident that, emotionally, it is still very much *present* tense for her. Through her eyes, she sees the attempt as 'dead and buried' for her husband, whereas she feels haunted by it and bombarded by regular reminders:

It will never fully go away. He has the ability to bury it so deeply that he doesn't think of it whereas it pings in my head when I hear any missing person, suicide, anything like that, I feel for those people. I do think that the likes of suicide awareness week does wonderful, wonderful work in raising awareness but never, ever, ever have I found anything that's – I think it's wonderful what they've done and they're also trying to get rid of the word 'committed', committed suicide, like, and I know I used it there but there isn't – there was never one article during suicide awareness day or week that ever thinks of any other impact on anyone else. There isn't [cries].

Tanya seems to relive the experience of her husband's attempt and all its associations when she is exposed to these reminders. At the heart of how Tanya experiences the world now is a sense of feeling like the forgotten one as everyone and everything seems to have moved on except her. In particular, she feels there is little if any focus given to significant others.

As was the case for both Alice and Tanya, the suicide attempt had many ripple effects for Carla, including distressing memories about growing up in an alcoholic household. She was intimately familiar with fear and tension while in her father's presence and these same feelings resurfaced while living with her husband for that short period after his attempt:

It certainly wasn't a pleasant atmosphere. It wasn't an aggressive atmosphere ... but yet, there was tension ... that I had previously experienced in my own family home as a young person. I was very aware that this tension was there and concerned as to how that tension impacted on the children, because I had a sense of how it impacted on me. I mean, we lived in a house where my father was an alcoholic and there was huge tension around his presence when he was there or imminently going to be there or whatever, and I felt that same tension. So that was a very familiar feeling to me and was loaded with fear and what-not, whatever I would have experienced when I was younger.

Carla was also concerned about whether her children were living through what she did during this time, something that also came up for Tanya regarding her own daughter. Another significant aspect of Carla's experience, in reaction to her husband's attempt, was her sense of obligation to not only leave her husband but the entire community that was connected to this marriage including in-laws, mutual friends, and even her own home:

I chose to leave all of that, so that was the marriage, the house, relationships and his family, apart from one whom I did stay connected to. So I chose that, as I saw it and I'm wondering now ... was that, in some sort of way, a punishment to myself ... oh, you're the one that left, so just suck it up, you've made this decision, you just have to take it on the chin.

Carla is perhaps suggesting here that she had to do what she thought was the honourable thing and fall on her own sword as 'punishment' for having instigated the demise of the marriage. There is probably some shame attached to her departure at a time that outsiders looking in would construe as his greatest hour of need, as well as to her decision to take the children away from their father. All of this coupled with the loss of a large part of her support network and her own home is likely to have deeply impacted Carla for some time.

The trauma of her husband's attempt forced Carla to confront many areas of her past that she thought she had either adequately buried or already processed. The one that was closest to her heart and rendered her the most fragile related to the child she gave up for adoption when she was in her late teens:

> I then would have addressed the issue of giving my daughter up for adoption, because that was a box that was sitting up on the shelf with a bow on it and, from an analytical perspective, I had sorted that one, but I hadn't connected with it on a feeling level at all until then. So, the counselling for that ... that took me to the next step which would have been taking that box down and walking that walk.

Carla speaks here about the part played by her husband's suicide attempt in forcing her to connect more with experiences in her life on an emotional rather than purely analytical level. She uses the metaphor of a 'box' with a 'bow' on it to perhaps portray her tendency to compartmentalize her life in the past. The suicide attempt completely disrupted this process, which created all kinds of emotional upheaval for her that would later be worked through in counselling.

Transcending death – Enhancing life

Rather than the suicide attempts defining their existence and dulling their sense of purpose, participants found that their experiences surpassed their expectations regarding the legacies of the attempts. This was neither expected nor planned by them. Participants described positive aspects of the legacies that were influential in their transformations to better versions of themselves. These included the ability to experience life to a heightened degree and no longer fear death, enhanced relationships with others, a greater sense of their inner strength, and the feeling that they were in greater touch with their spiritual selves.

Carla's view of what 'normal' is for her now starkly contrasts her life prior to her husband's suicide attempt. The attempt was the final nail in the coffin for the relationship and heralded a difficult but ultimately satisfying journey of self-discovery:

> I suppose, finding myself and my own voice ... when you join all those things up together, there's no one particular thing, but really being free to be who I've become, or being free to start the journey of finding who I am, who I was and who I am now has been a long journey and a very interesting journey and a very empowering journey, and would have started with stopping the relationship.

Her conclusion here is that resources such as friendships, counselling, and her openness to face any 'skeletons' from her past enabled her to transcend the trauma of her husband's suicide attempt and to enhance her relationship with her 'true' self. Carla's newfound sense of freedom to be herself and to develop her own voice reflects the transformation she has undergone as a result of her experience.

This freedom also rechannelled her energy into motherhood, a role that she relished but at times felt she didn't live up to because of the demands of her marriage:

I've always said I was a better mother as a result of it than had I stayed in the marriage. I think I would have ended up, well, I don't know, but I think I would have probably ended up either an alcoholic or depending on something to support me in the supporting of him and that the children would have gotten lost somewhere in the middle, that if I had to stay focusing on that relationship, he would have gotten so much that it would have been to the detriment of myself and my children and, in not being in the relationship … I can't say it's his fault … I think it's not being in the relationship I was free to be what I wanted which was a mum, part of me wanted to be that.

Life for Carla now means renewed self-esteem and a greater confidence to be the mother she has always wanted to be. Having experienced the suffering that followed his attempt, she recognizes that where she is now both emotionally and psychologically is infinitely better than where she would have been had she remained in the marriage. This, of course, can only have positive implications for her children and her relationship with them in the future. It is evident that Carla has invested time and energy into her reflections about this life-changing experience and its implications for how she wishes to relate to the world going forward:

The importance of keeping a sense of self within a relationship, within any relationship, being watchful of where the relationship is, I mean, is there a very strong parental person/role within a relationship? ... I've experienced people who ... there's a strong Mammy thing of mammying people ... to be careful of that, because then there's a lack of equality, you're not two adults in a relationship, you're a parent and a child relationship. I don't allow things anymore to ... if I've an issue with something, I look at it. If there's a feeling ... I always look at it and say, 'What's this about?' Feelings, sorry, I never mentioned feelings, did I? Nobody should ever ignore their feelings and we subdue them so much.

Carla's transformation has culminated in an enhanced sense of self, clearer boundaries, and the ability to face issues head on. Crucially, she now gives herself permission to feel regardless of what comes to the surface.

In contrast to the other participants, Margaret was markedly positive about the long-term ramifications of her husband's attempt. She would have preferred them to have been a closer couple but she was quite philosophical about accepting the things that she could not change. Of particular note is her post-attempt awareness of a deep well of untapped resources already within her, which actually enhanced her life:

> *Life after was better for me than it was before in a strange way. I was able to – I had the ability to make life better, you know, I realized that I could do it.*

Margaret's new-found empowerment created a sea change in that she began to assert her needs and to develop a life independent of her husband, something that was long overdue:

> *It's made me a much stronger thinking person ... I would always sort of say ... 'Can I have the car to go wherever?' ... whereas then I set about getting my own car and being independent and not having to go to ... that depressive level maybe, if one person is living in a depressing sort of state doesn't mean that the other person has to join them, and I felt I can rise above this ... and ... that took steps ... tiny steps ... not maybe always ideal, but it was my way of surviving.*

Margaret learned that if someone in her life was in psychological despair, she was not obliged to stay in that depressive place with them and that, through tentative steps forward, she could transcend her husband's experience.

Margaret's experience forced her to face the possibility that she could be widowed at some point in the future and this afforded her a rare opportunity to be exposed to the loss of her husband, albeit from a safe vantage point:

I think probably, so as if it ever happened again, I would be prepared, I would be more capable of dealing with it. I would ... have myself set up to probably be able to live independently, that it wouldn't be such a big blow if he did commit suicide, I would be ready ... maybe.

Margaret's growing empowerment is evident here in her ability to visualize being on her own. Set against the backdrop of living with the uncertainty of whether he would attempt suicide again, her greatest resource, were he to do so, would be to have the fundamentals in place to live a healthy life in his absence.

An important part of her journey has also entailed relinquishing the illusion that she is personally responsible for whether he lives or dies:

You then figure out that you can't run after somebody watching them and you have to be able to sort of block out that section, that if they go out the door, that it's their choice where they go or what they do, that you carry on with life. You have to develop your own life that doesn't involve living in that circle all the time.

Margaret uses the image of a circle to perhaps represent the merry-go-round of caretaking that she has endured over the years because of his fluctuating mental health and alcoholism. It may also represent her feeling trapped in a cycle over which she had no sense of control and from which she could not escape. Either way, both the circle and the cycle have been broken and Margaret has become acquainted with the spiritual side of her with which she was unfamiliar:

> *I've learned to trust in maybe a higher authority than me ... accept that you don't control what's laid out for you in life and you just accept it, whatever it throws at you ... I'm not hugely religious, but I would be – I suppose religion does play a part in it, yes. Faith is a good ... I think people who don't have a focus point in their life, it must be very hard, whatever religion ...*

There's a sense here that Margaret has personal contentment in her life now. Perhaps, she is implying that she is happy *in spite of* what may be going on for her husband at any given time. It seems that this woman's life experience, especially since the suicide attempt, has created a more grounded mentality and, with it, more realistic expectations of life.

Although the bond in the relationship for Tanya, Carla and Margaret has been irrevocably damaged to varying degrees, Evan's story feels worlds apart. He believes his wife's attempt has brought him closer to her in a way that is unrecognizable to anything previously in the relationship:

> *I think ... the whole relationship has evolved into something that never was in the beginning ... The two people that got married were completely alien to me*

now, to the two people that are here now. Now that's
probably the same in most marriages because of time
and all the rest of it, but I think for all that's gone on and
all that we've been through together ...

Evan describes both himself and his wife objectively as if he is an outside party looking inwards. He uses the term 'alien' which evokes unfamiliarity, the supernatural, and, perhaps, the spiritual dimension. He acknowledges that change is par for the course in all relationships but suggests that both he and his wife, in particular, have transformed to an extent *far* beyond the typical range of experience.

It is clear that Evan has a greater self-respect since the suicide attempt and, indeed, a greater mutual respect as he admires all the 'wonderful things' she has gone on to do with her life. He talks about the attempt as a moment of 'rebirth' for his wife. In many ways, however, it has marked a rebirth for both of them individually and as a couple:

Probably better than it's ever been. I think I certainly
love the person I'm with now much more than I loved
the person I married. I certainly love them differently
... but certainly ... it's definitely two people individually
leading ... or living a collective life, if that makes sense.
There's no expectations of each other.

It strikes as quite a startling admission to say you love your spouse *much* more than when you first married. This probably reflects, however, the sheer level of impact and the depth of trans-formation Evan has experienced on the basis of the suicide attempt.

Evan mentioned that, in hindsight, they needed someone to stir the 'murky water' so that positive change could occur. His wife's attempt certainly achieved this to the extent that it stirred something up in their relationship dynamic also:

> *It's funny because our individuality has acknowledged itself, it's very present in the sense that ... in a lovely way. So that's basically where we're at, at the minute, you know. It's all good, has all its problems, still has all its problems and all the rest of it, but it's all good.*

This may suggest a co-dependent relationship prior to the attempt which has since rectified itself. The metamorphosis and rebirth that followed the attempt are juxtaposed with all the 'normal' ups and downs of a happy marriage.

Evan also had a rather philosophical outlook on his experience of his wife's attempt. He described it as a 'massive journey' and akin to one train crash after another. He was positive overall, however, about how it has shaped him as a person:

> *It's taken the edges off, and rounded me more ... I think, to get them edges off ... you know when you look at stones and you go ... 'that must have been in a river' ... I think it takes nature to take them edges off. I don't think you can grind them off, or rub them down, I think they have to wear away, you know and the whole process has definitely done that for me.*

Evan likens himself to a stone that has become a softer version of itself through time and experience. He suggests that aspects of his personality such as patience, empathy, and tolerance have evolved in response to the extreme pressures he felt during the ebb and flow of the experience. He sees this evolution as something that cannot be manufactured or rushed, but, like a river, it follows its own course in its own time.

Witnessing his wife being very close to death and all that ensued, Evan began to reflect on his own mortality, which was a revelation for him:

For me and my life, it has absolutely ... here's one for you, I don't know if I ever feared death, but I certainly don't now.

Evan is uncertain here whether he was ever afraid of death, but he is now convinced that her suicide attempt extinguished any remnants of fear in him. His achievement of greater ease with the circle of life and his acceptance of death had an inextricable spiritual dimension to it according to Evan:

I'd be spiritual, but I wouldn't be religious. But that was definitely a spiritual journey without a shadow of a doubt for both of us and I think that if you're really lucky, you get to grasp that, you get to realize that ... and I think we've been really lucky. On a selfish note, I wouldn't change a thing [laughs].

Significantly, Evan communicates that the journey is one that was made *together* with his wife and, therefore, enhanced their relationship. He implies that not all couples who go through this may grasp this important spiritual dimension of the experience. In fact, it seems it has been so life-changing for him that he is, in many respects, thankful for it.

Conclusion: transformations for better, for worse

Findings suggest that the impact of a partner's suicide attempt is transformational for individuals and followed both negative and positive trajectories. Analysis has revealed that transformation occurred for participants as a result of the trauma they suffered during these life-changing experiences. Their shattered assumptions manifested in the midst of shock, feelings of hurt, betrayal, and desperation to comprehend what had happened. All the while, they continued to meet life's obligations. The participants' transformative experiences continued apace with the complex adjustment in the wake of the attempts, their navigation through self-blame and blame from others (both perceived and explicit), and their development of ways to counter the torment. The impact on partners left a permanent, transformative legacy that compelled them to both confront unresolved adverse childhood experiences and embrace new growth within themselves, their relationships, and their outlook on life.

PART II

IMPACT AND
RECOVERY
FOR PARTNERS

CHAPTER 5

Changing the landscape on attempted suicide

Introduction

Suicide, an act in which one ... destroys one's self and which challenges the fundamental meaning of life, is perhaps the most lonely and most impersonal act that can be performed by a human being ... There are few other acts that so profoundly affect others.'

Talseth, Gilje and Norberg, 2001, p. 249

The evidence offered in Part I of this book in many ways speaks for itself in terms of highlighting how human beings worldwide have either minimized the lived experience of partners and significant others or been wholly unaware of the tumultuous ripple effect a suicide attempt can have socially. It is clear that the experience transforms the world of the partner in many different ways. Chapter 6 assimilates the insights from participants into concrete ways so that we can really start to understand just how incredibly transformative the event actually is for them. Prior to this, however, it may prove useful to offer more context by taking a look at what was known about attempted suicide and its impact on others up until the present study was undertaken. In this way, an even deeper appreciation for the potential therapeutic gains for partners, 'other' significant others, and even the relationship between the partner and suicide attempter can be developed.

Most of the research in the area of suicide has, so far, not shown any real interest in hearing from the partners and significant others of those who have attempted suicide. In the recent past, researchers have paid increased attention to the relatives of those who have attempted suicide but really only to learn more about the attempters themselves rather than to gain a deeper understanding of the relatives' own personal experiences. While gaining a deeper understanding of the suicide attempter's experience is, of course, vital, the experience of significant others, the partner in particular, has tended to be ignored. My focus has always been on the personal impact on partners specifically, but you will notice as you read on that studies have tended for the most part to target a broad spectrum of participants within the same study – parents, adult children, siblings, friends, as well as partners, with the general aim of furthering our understanding of suicide and burden of care for families.

Attempted suicide in the context of significant others

Erwin Stengel (1956), an Austrian-born scholar at the Institute of Psychiatry in London, highlighted that, in 1941, the estimated global 'attempted suicide' to 'completed suicide' ratio was thought to be in the region of 6:1. It is frightening to note, then, that today, attempted suicide is up to 20+ times more frequent than completed suicide (World Health Organization, 2021), with an attempted suicide probably occurring every one to two seconds somewhere in the world. The World Health Organization (WHO) reports that, globally, approximately 800,000 people die by suicide on an annual basis but had actually predicted that, by the year 2020, approximately 1.5 million individuals worldwide would die by suicide (WHO, 1999), and this figure was not taking into consideration the potential fallout of the global pandemic that began in late 2019. Therefore, if 20 times more people attempted suicide as per the estimates, then over 30 million individuals worldwide would have experienced a suicide attempt. If this is applied to Irish figures, since 421 individuals ('provisional', year of registration data) died by suicide in 2019 (National Office for Suicide Prevention, 2021), then approximately 8420 individuals would have attempted suicide in the Republic of Ireland in that year. Applied to England and Wales, the estimated number of suicide attempts in 2019 would amount to almost 114,000 (Office for National Statistics, 2020). According to the American Foundation for Suicide Prevention (AFSP, 2021), there was an estimated 1.38 million suicide attempts in 2019 in the US.

Annette Beautrais, a New Zealand suicidologist, estimates that up to six individuals are directly affected by a suicide (Beautrais, 2004). In Ireland, however, a national service for those bereaved by suicide, *Console* (now part of Pieta House), estimated that a minimum of twelve people are affected by suicide (Tierney, 2011). If both of these estimates are applied to the population of suicide attempters, then there may be a population of between approximately 50,000 and 100,000 individuals affected by a suicide attempt in Ireland each year, a population of between 700,000 and 1.3 million individuals affected within England and Wales, and between eight and sixteen million individuals potentially impacted across the US. These figures reflect the staggering number of people whose personal lived experiences are overshadowed by the suicide attempts of their loved ones.

Attempted suicide and significant others: being met as an informant/caregiver vs being met as a person

The little research I have come across that pays any attention to significant others has done so with respect to their role as either the 'informant' who provides researchers with information to improve the well-being of suicide attempters or the 'caregiver' who is required to maintain strategies to help care for suicidal relatives. This really highlights the pressure placed on the significant others because of society's response to this life crisis. Some of the symptoms a significant other might experience while caring for an actively suicidal individual have been recorded but no concerted effort, until now, has ever really been made to capture a deeper personal account of the experience from their perspective.

Research on attempted suicide that also makes reference to other family members first surfaced in the early 1960s, but it has been rarely touched on since then. The earliest research I came across was a 1964 American unpublished study by Hattem (Harris, 1966) that actually suggested that partners of those who were suicidal had somehow *driven* the individual to perform the act! Harris (1966) embarked on a follow-up study to ascertain the impact of maintaining or ending the relationship on further suicidal behaviours. Fifteen of the original twenty individuals from Hattem's study took part in a structured interview. Of the eight individuals who remained with their partner, four continued to exhibit suicidal behaviour. The other seven individuals who separated from their partner exhibited no further suicidal behaviour. Both researchers, however, only got half the story as they gathered information from the suicidal individuals but not from partners. Thus, this explanation is not only grossly oversimplified but sets up a culture of blame for someone's suicidal behaviour.

A later Swedish study (Wolk-Wasserman, 1986) found that, of the 70 'significant others' of 37 suicide attempt patients admitted to hospital, the vast majority of significant others grasped they were suicidal but responded with almost total silence. More recent research (Deisenhammer, Huber, Kemmler, Weiss and Hinterhuber, 2007) suggests that individuals discharged from psychiatric hospital are at greater risk of suicide just after discharge with 47.7 per cent dying by suicide within one month of discharge (n = 665). Thus, it stands to reason that both hospital and mental health professionals' priority is to mobilize immediate family members (including partners) to ensure the survival of those who have previously attempted suicide. The personal impact on the partner is thereby lost in the midst of this life-or-death crisis.

It was not until 1998 that Swedish researchers Magne-Ingvar and Öjehagen (1999a) first recorded the well-being of significant others, just under a third of whom were current partners of the suicide attempters. The rest comprised former partners, parents, adult children, siblings, and friends.

Of the 81 significant others (SOs) contacted by telephone over a 16-month period:

- Of the SOs who had provided emotional or practical support to the patients, before and following the attempts, 57 per cent reported this to have been a significant weight on them. In addition, they felt that the pressure was worse if the patients were living with a psychiatric disorder.
- On finding out about the suicide attempt, 75 per cent of SOs reported feelings of worry, upset, and shock.
- On exploration of their own health, 16 per cent of SOs reported feeling physically unwell.
- Approximately 25 per cent communicated sleep, mood, and/or appetite difficulties.
- Other personal problems *on top of* the demands of care were reported by 41 per cent.
- Fifty-three per cent reported an interest in engaging in counselling *conjointly* with the patients while 37

per cent only wanted individual counselling. This may indicate the tendency for SOs to prioritize the welfare of their partners rather than their own welfare.

The researchers contacted the same relatives and friends one year later (Magne-Ingvar and Öjehagen, 1999b) and found that over three-quarters of them worried that the patient would engage in further deliberate self-harm following the initial suicide attempt. Approximately 60 per cent of SOs reported at least one of the following symptoms:

- worry
- tiredness
- headache
- irritability
- downheartedness
- epigastric pain
- disrupted sleep
- tension
- hopelessness
- anxiety.

What is really significant for partners in comparison to other significant others is that partners reported less social supports, lingering questions about the suicide attempts, unsatisfactory well-being, and a greater need to seek out individual professional support.

Another Swedish study, carried out a number of years later (Östman and Kjellin, 2002), explored the experience of stigma for relatives of individuals with mental illness. The study reinforced the findings of the aforementioned studies in that spouses of individuals with mental illness, in comparison to other relatives, were found to show a higher rate of difficulties within the relationships, a higher rate of mental health issues and suicidal ideation ... and a greater wish that they had never met their spouses. The same researchers were charting the difficulty of caring for those at risk of suicide in 1988, 1991, and 1997. Östman, Wallsten, and Kjellin (2005) interviewed nearly 500 relatives of patients admitted to psychiatric care both voluntarily and involuntarily, which included parents, spouses, adult children, siblings as well as non-relatives. They found that approximately one-third of the relatives had concerns about the patients making suicide attempts and reported their own mental health difficulties. Relatives living with the patients demonstrated greater distress than those not living with the patients. In addition, spouses displayed more negative psychological impact overall than the other relatives. Spouses more often felt less inclined to socialize with others and experienced feelings of isolation as a result. They also tended to be far more involved in in-patient treatment and had to give up work more often to prioritize the care of their partners. This research once again highlights the pressure that relatives can experience to take responsibility in managing their loved one's mental health condition, and the fear that the individual *might* make a suicide attempt. It didn't, however, paint a detailed picture of what it is like to live with a loved one during and following their suicide attempt. All of these studies spotlight the potential negative impact that a suicide attempt can have on partners and significant others but they provide only a snapshot of their symptoms rather than an in-depth understanding of the *personal* impact on partners and its meaning for their everyday lives.

A very limited amount of information is available about a patient's home life after discharge from psychiatric hospital, as is the case with the experience of partners and significant others. Sun and colleagues later explored both the family carer's and ex-patient's perceptions of their home lives and the provision of care at home (Sun, Long, Huang and Huang, 2008). They interviewed thirteen individuals who had attempted suicide and two who had experienced suicidal thoughts. They also interviewed fifteen family members. The suicidal individuals had just been discharged from one of two Taiwanese hospitals. The fifteen 'carers' were either partners, parents, siblings, or adult children. The interviews revealed that family members experienced worry and a heavy feeling of responsibility following patient discharge, as they feared that the individuals would attempt suicide when not under their supervision. The researchers later described this as 'guarding the person day and night'.

The degree of closeness within the relationships was also found to impact the home environments, with pre-existing closeness positively influencing communication and poorer relationships resulting in greater distancing between members. The main emotions that surfaced for carers were tiredness, anger, stress, fear, anguish, and numbness. The stigma associated with the suicide attempt was also felt by family members due to the particularly negative view Chinese culture takes on suicide. This stigma is a common theme shared across most cultures and continents to varying degrees which leaves its mark on all concerned.

In 2009, Sun and colleagues wrote about the need for family members to co-operate in the care of those who had attempted suicide (Sun, Long, Huang and Chiang, 2009). They suggested that this co-operation should include responsibilities such as:

- constantly checking in on how suicidal their relative is
- protecting their relative from self-harm
- promoting daily activities to encourage their recovery
- creating as nurturing an environment as possible
- ensuring that all that can be done to improve the individual's mental health is put into practice.

It is clear from this list that what is involved in this so-called 'co-operation' from family caregivers is substantial. There is a clear expectation by society that they take on the enormous task of ensuring the safety and recovery of suicidal relatives with any emotional or physical costs to family members deemed of little or no importance. In fact, the same authors wrote about the importance of educating family members about suicide in 2013 and in 2014, describing how family members could create the best conditions for healing following a loved one's suicide attempt. In my view, an important piece of the jigsaw is missing, namely, the examination of the personal impact on family members especially partners.

Another study that explored the support needs of family members caring for a suicidal person (McLaughlin, McGowan, Kernohan and O'Neill, 2016) acknowledged the loneliness and isolation that participants experienced, but again its emphasis was on highlighting ways in which they as 'carers' could be better supported in supporting their suicidal relatives. Eighteen individuals were interviewed, seven of whom had already experienced the death through suicide of a parent or sibling, and eleven were living with a relative displaying suicidal behaviour (suicidal ideation, self-harm and/or attempted suicide). The support needs that emerged from the interviews comprised:

1. practical support, respite, and advice from healthcare staff
2. acknowledgement and a sense of inclusion
3. someone to turn to, and
4. consistency in the support they received from staff.

This study is clearly very much a step in the right direction in terms of exposing the blatant lack of information-sharing between the professions and family carers, particularly where patients are over eighteen years of age and issues of confidentiality get in the way of optimum care provision.

More recently, Hvidkaer *et al.* (2020) have confirmed that there is very little empirical data about the impact on individuals who have been exposed to the suicide attempt of someone in their life. Their online survey accessing over 6000 Danish citizens examined possible correlations between exposure to an attempted suicide, well-being and suicidal ideation. Almost one-quarter of the respondents reported having been exposed to an attempt, and scored lower on general well-being and higher on suicidal ideation themselves.

In addition, they were more severely impacted if the suicide attempt was made by a close relative. Of significance also, was the finding that half of those exposed to the attempt felt they had not received adequate support in the aftermath. This finding highlights in literal terms the 50:50 chance of being sufficiently supported in the wake of a suicide attempt.

So what conclusions can we draw?

The majority of the studies I have highlighted above confirm how central family members are to the safety and recovery of those who are suicidal or attempt suicide. It is quire clear, however, based on the personal experiences of partners depicted in Part I that there is a gross assumption made by society, including those in both the medical and the mental health professions, that partners are physically and emotionally able or, indeed, motivated to take on such considerable responsibility. In fact, there is some evidence suggesting that significant others coping with an actively suicidal loved one are actually at greater risk of suicide themselves (Gustafsson, 1999). Yet it is significant others, partners in particular, who are identified as the main caregivers! The following Chapter illuminates the *context* of a partner's experience after an attempted suicide, beyond the position of caregiver.

CHAPTER 6

Charting the transformative impact on partners

Introduction

The interviews with partners were conducted with a view to exploring their lived experience of being in the post-attempt relationship and to examine the meaning that partners attributed to the suicide attempt and their outlook on life after the attempt.

The study revealed a transformative impact on participants on the basis of their loved one's suicide attempt. This transformation manifested in both positive and adverse ways. The experience had a traumatizing impact on them represented by the first theme, 'It put nearly ten years on my life': suffering the trauma of the attempt. They experienced recurrent shock associated with the event, 'It's a shock that comes in waves', and feeling like 'the walking wounded', experiencing raw pain and extreme adverse feelings towards their partner, all the while honouring practical and financial obligations. Their strong desire to be relieved from ambiguity was denoted by their 'desperate search for answers'. A significant aspect of the second theme 'It shifted the whole world on its axis': adjusting in the wake of the attempt, was their own efforts to gain insight into whom or what was responsible for the suicide attempt and what if anything they could have done to prevent it. Participants consequently found themselves playing 'the blame game'. They also developed 'strategies for self-preservation' as a means of 'countering the torment', both emotional and psychological. For some this encompassed renegotiation of boundaries and, for others, a complete disengagement from their partner. The final theme, 'It never ever goes away': the legacy of the attempt, represents 'What lies beneath', which arose for participants in terms of the attempt altering their perception of the relationship and which they kept private. The attempt also brought to the surface adverse childhood memories for some and deterioration in physical health for others, which have lingered to the present day. Participants also had the experience of 'transcending death – enhancing life' as a legacy, illustrated by growth across a number of domains including personal relationships and outlook on life.

This chapter aims to make sense of the research findings from the interviews shared in Part I by contextualizing them within extant literature, both empirical and theoretical, and in so doing exploring how the findings build on what we already know. It was found that participants' experiences were underpinned by multiple traumas, which caused a permanent and profound transformation of their assumptive world. Literature on trauma theory and the phenomenon of complex trauma, will therefore, be examined in more depth. Findings also suggest that participants experienced a transformation of their 'psychological family'. Literature will be explored more closely on a significant aspect of ambiguous loss theory known as boundary ambiguity. Participants in this study all experienced a transformation in their perception of the quality of their attachment relationship pre- and post-suicide attempt and, therefore, it was deemed prudent to examine the literature on attachment theory and the implications of affectional bond violations. Finally, findings highlighted that the majority of participants were not only resilient in the wake of their partner's suicide attempt, but experienced suffering-induced transformation in personal strength, spirituality, outlook on life, and relating to others. Literature on post-traumatic growth theory will be examined in the light of this. The following sections provide an overview of the impact on 'significant others' based on the study findings, and offers an in-depth treatment of the concept of 'transformation'.

Impact on 'significant others'

It has been estimated (Beautrais, 2004) that up to six 'significant others' could be impacted by a suicide, whereas Tierney (2011) gave a less conservative estimate at a minimum of twelve individuals. It was assumed that a similar number of significant others would be affected by a serious suicide attempt. This, however, did *not* seem to be borne out in my exploration with the five participants. 'Significant others' (parents, grown-up children, siblings, close friends) were informed on a need-to-know basis only and with some of the participants no one other than the attempter and their partner were ever aware that the attempt had occurred. Although a 'completed' suicide would have signified an actual physical death and some degree of public mourning and ritual that could not be avoided, the attempted suicide of a partner turned out to be an incredibly lonely journey for participants, with their grief very much hidden and disenfranchised. For the in-laws of participants who were informed of their partner's suicide attempt, it seemed that their priority was to figure out 'what to do with him/her'. In other words, they were motivated to ensure the immediate physical safety of their brother, sister, son or daughter, preferably back under the care of his or her partner. From the perspective of the partners who participated in this study, however, the *long-* rather than the short-term impact was experienced by them.

Understanding 'transformation' and its relevance for partners

The main thrust of the findings saw participants experiencing *profound* change in various domains. For some the profound change manifested in how they saw themselves, for others how they saw the world and people within it, and for others still how they saw their partner and their relationship. Most participants, however, experienced profound change in all domains. As the average length of time since the suicide attempt at interview was 10.5 years, all participants viewed these changes as not only permanent but ongoing.

'Change', however, does not adequately capture the depth or breadth of how participants experienced their partner's suicide attempt. One participant talked about her 'world shifting on its axis', another talked about 're-birth' and 'metamorphosis'. I postulate, therefore, that participants experienced 'transformations' of various kinds on the basis of their partner's attempts. The literature within psychotherapy tends to conceptualize transformation with either positive *or* negative connotations. For example, Bray (2013) offers a perspective from transpersonal psychology, the interface between human beings and spirituality, which describes transformation as an expansion of one's worldview, consciousness, and psyche. On the other hand, Neimeyer (2000) suggests that in loss, one can never fully resolve one's loss but is actually permanently transformed by it. The following authors, however, provide conceptualizations that offer scope for viewing transformation from both positive and negative perspectives. Tedeschi and Calhoun (2004) offer a more neutral definition of transformation in the context of trauma, describing it as 'a qualitative change in functioning' (p.4). Within social research, 'transformation' is portrayed as:

the process of moving from one state of being to another: this may apply *inter alia* to abilities, awareness, knowledge, consciousness, environment, social status, fortune or well-being. (Harvey, 2019)

Taylor (2012) offers a view of transformation within humanistic psychology, positing that it can not only manifest over a period of time but also entail 'a very abrupt shift to a completely different state of being', with experiences being 'sometimes so powerful that they lead to permanent change of being, and even a permanent state of enlightenment'. (Taylor, 2012, p. 32)

Harvey (2019) further explicates the meaning of transformation for the individual and the far-reaching implications it inevitably has for their world view and within the context of relating to self and other:

> Transformation is about a fundamental change of form (and often functioning). It is much more than adjustment or repositioning; and implies more than reform, reawakening or reconsideration. It is closer to revolution in meaning and requires a fundamental re-evaluation and reconstruction. (Harvey, 2019)

Daszko and Sheinberg (2017) also offer a view of transformation through an occupational psychology lens that is akin to the Greek term 'metanoia' meaning 'beyond the mind'. This suggests that transformation considers affective, somatic, spiritual, as well as cognitive experience:

> It's an idea of stretching or pushing beyond the boundaries with which we normally think and feel. It means a profound change in mind, a radical revision, a transformation of our whole mental process, a paradigm shift. (Daszko and Sheinberg 2017, p. 1)

They, too, see transformation as qualitatively profound, creating shifts at a fundamental level, is uncharted territory, and ultimately developing into something new that never was before. Like Harvey (2019) they operationalize it as a fluid process encompassing a multitude of actions rather than an immediate or abrupt shift:

> Transformation occurs through ... continual questioning, challenging, exploration, discovery, evaluation, testing ... beginning with the realization or revelation that the [person]'s current thinking is incomplete, limiting, flawed, or even worse – destructive. In transformation, there is no known destination, and the journey has never been travelled before. It is uncertain and unpredictable. It embraces new learning and taking actions based on the new discoveries. (Daszko and Sheinberg, 2017, p. 4)

According to Ebert (2010), what sets 'transformation' apart from simple 'change' is that transformation is neither linear nor foreseeable. In summary, then, what participants experienced in the wake of their partner's suicide attempt was a fundamental shift or re-evaluation of being and functioning in response to revelations that permeated multiple modalities, and, therefore was by definition a 'transformation'.

Transformation generally has connotations of encompassing a positive trajectory. However, participants had experiences that suggested transformation existing on a continuum between 'adverse transformation' and 'positive transformation'. In addition, for the majority of participants paradoxically both adverse *and* positive transformation occurred, that is, it was a case of *both/and* rather than *either/or*.

Transformation of the 'assumptive world'

'Adverse transformation' occurred for participants as a result of the trauma of their partner's suicide attempt. Rather than experiencing acute stress that was transient in nature, participants' experience comprised multiple traumas manifesting from the trauma of: (1) exposure to the attempt; (2) the suicide attempt triggering previous childhood trauma (for some participants); (3) ambiguous loss within the partnership; and (4) attachment injury, all of which had far-reaching consequences.

Participants' initial engagement with the suicide attempt, subsequent exposure to events in the hospital setting, their desperate search for answers, the shock that visited them in waves, and their overall sense of struggling to survive it, all contributed to participants' experience of it as *extra*-ordinary, far beyond the normal range of experience. Fosha's (2006) definition of the transformative potential of trauma captures perfectly, the impact of the event for participants:

> Trauma is the *definitum* of quantum transformation: in one fell swoop, everything changes. Nothing is ever the same again. (Fosha, 2006, p. 569)

The personal impact for participants in the present study

was found to be very similar to the impact described by individuals in Sands and Tennant's (2010) study who were actually bereaved by suicide. As in the present study themes connected with 'staying alive', 'culpability and motive', 'why' issues connected with responsibility, blame, guilt, confusion, and failure, and 'reorienting in a shattered world' manifested for those who were survivors of a relative's completed suicide. This has potentially significant implications in terms of assessment and psychotherapeutic intervention for the partners of attempted suicide, which are discussed in Chapter 7.

The trauma of a partner's suicide attempt is transformational in that it tears apart the individual's long-held assumptions and core beliefs about how the world is *supposed* to work. Janoff-Bulman (1992) posits that people essentially maintain psychological and emotional balance by believing in certain illusions such as the world is a good and meaningful place. When they experience a trauma, a dissonance is created between their 'assumptive world' and their reality:

> Life as it was and even as it has become is difficult to maintain on a day-to-day basis, and individuals are forced to reconcile themselves to the realities of shattered assumptive worlds. (Bray, 2013, p. 899)

An intricate part of this frightening experience for individuals is the subsequent challenge to 'transform' their now obsolete template of the world into a new template that takes account of 'non-ordinary knowledge and experiences' (Bray, 2013, p.899).

Fosha's (2006) understanding of trauma as transformation is further explicated by the American Psychiatric Association's (APA's) operationalization of trauma as 'exposure [direct or indirect] to actual or threatened death ... to a close family member or close friend ... or experiences first-hand repeated or extreme exposure to aversive details of the traumatic event' (APA, 2013, para. 2).

This study is the first ever to recognize the impact of an attempted suicide as traumatic for partners. Until now, this very vulnerable group have been prioritized as caregivers with little or no priority given to their psychological or emotional welfare. It is vital, therefore, to highlight the potential that their lived experience could fall within the realm of clinically significant trauma. Participants in this study were adversely transformed in being and functioning as a result of both witnessing their partner's suicide attempt in progress and later witnessing the, at times, aggressive attempts to save their life. The genesis of transformation for participants occurred across four domains in which the trauma manifested: re-experiencing; avoidance; negative cognitions and mood; and arousal.

Re-experiencing for participants was described variously as the suicide attempt 'pinging' spontaneously in their head on a frequent basis, and experiencing the distress from it 'never going away'. Some participants avoided talking with their partner or others about the experience but they were unable to avoid their partners who were constant reminders of the suicide attempt, or places associated with the attempt for that matter as most took place within their own home. Some participants refused to have their partner return to the family home when they were discharged from hospital but eventually they returned. With regard to negative cognitions and mood, participants talked about feeling helpless and a sense of hopelessness. They were acutely aware of feeling to blame or of blaming others and experienced a desire to withdraw from others. For some participants the experience was so traumatic that they cannot recall parts of it to this day. Arousal for participants manifested in anger toward their partner, and in sleeplessness and hyper-vigilance for fear of another suicide attempt occurring 'on their watch'. This further added to the complexity of participant's unique trauma as there was an element of exposure to 'compassion fatigue' in the midst of living through the event, which is a form of stress as a result of being exposed to the emotional suffering of others (Figley, 1995). Both 'fight' and 'flight' were a feature of participant's trauma. 'Flight' constituted avoidance behaviours and 'fight' constituted behaviours such as arguing with hospital staff, refusal to leave the counselling service until their partner was seen, challenging partners to take their own lives in moments of exasperation, and physically removing a partner from a psychiatric hospital when they perceived the care to be inadequate.

The domains described above converge very much with those articulated in the diagnostic literature for post-traumatic stress (WHO, 1992; APA, 2013). A significant divergence, however, is that, for participants in this study, they are among a very small proportion of the world's population who have been exposed to an extraordinary phenomenon in which both primary traumatic stress and compassion fatigue (secondary traumatic stress) featured for them. Participants were not only traumatized by their partner's suicide attempt but continued to be exposed to their partner, the source of their trauma, when she or he returned home. Participants felt the strain of compassion and pity towards their partner, but at the same time were motivated to be hypervigilant around them in order to minimize the likelihood of being exposed to further trauma should their partner attempt suicide for a second time. For some participants, therefore, disengaging from their partner (either fully or partially) may have constituted an avoidant defence mechanism so as to ensure their own psychological and emotional 'survival'. The phenomenon of concomitant primary trauma and compassion fatigue is complex insofar as a traumatized individual has a complex relationship to the source of their trauma, their partner in this case, in which they are at once compelled to ensure their welfare and repelled by them in order to minimize further trauma. In other circumstances where trauma features, avoidance behaviours are an adaptive response to ensure survival. In this context, this intuitive response is neither personally nor socially sanctioned.

Transformative activation of memory and physiology

In addition to participant's experience of their partner's suicide attempt as traumatic, a number of them felt that it triggered unresolved trauma from childhood which exacerbated their circumstances. Three of the five participants shared experiences of: intrusive distressing memories regarding childhood physical, sexual, and emotional abuse; a parent's tragic and sudden death as a result of a road traffic accident; a father's alcoholism; and early traumatic loss as a result of giving a first-born child up for adoption. These memories inevitably negatively impacted participant's emotional and psychological equilibrium, which in turn reduced their ability to withstand the trauma of their partner's suicide attempt. Cumulatively, trauma experienced as a result of the suicide attempt, compassion fatigue, and reactivation of childhood trauma, made participants particularly vulnerable to developing mental health difficulties. These all had a transformative effect on participants, permanently re-evaluating assumptions they had developed about self, other and the world.

A number of meta-analytical studies reinforce this point of just how significant our early exposure to adversity is for coping with adversity in *later* years. Brewin, Andrews and Valentine (2000) looked at risk factors for post-traumatic stress disorder (PTSD) in trauma-exposed adults and found that previous exposure to trauma, degree of childhood adversity, reported childhood abuse, and family psychiatric history were among the strongest predictors. Furthermore, greater severity of trauma, less access to social supports, and concurrent stressors increased the likelihood of developing PTSD. Likewise, Ozer, Best, Lipsey and Weiss' (2008) meta-analysis of predictors of PTSD or of its symptoms in adults found that among the predictors established were prior trauma; prior psychological adjustment, family history of mental health difficulties, social support post-trauma, and peri-trauma emotional responses.

Both of the aforementioned meta-analyses found that prior trauma, poor social supports, and adverse family history all contributed to poor coping with adversity in later life. All of these predictors were found to feature in the lived experience of some of the participants in the current study (that is, childhood sexual abuse, living with the knowledge of the suicide attempt in isolation, and a family history of adversity such as parental separation and alcoholism). Another aspect of a participant's reactivation of childhood trauma is Freud's psychoanalytical construct of *Nachträglichkeit*, otherwise known as deferred action, retroaction, or afterwardness. *Nachträglichkeit* is defined by Freud as 'a memory which is repressed which has only become a trauma *after the event*' (cited in Laplanche, 1976, p. 41). A prime example in the context of the current study occurred for a participant when, on thinking about the potential traumatic impact on her young daughter had her partner actually killed himself, she recalled her own experience at eight years of age of police coming to their home to inform the family that her father had been killed in a road traffic accident. This had the effect of transforming an otherwise relatively sombre memory into a traumatic one. Thus, aspects of the present experience for some participants had the effect of assessing aspects of previous experience as traumatic, *after* the fact.

Adverse physiological transformation was another significant aspect for some of the participants in this study who noted general deterioration in their own physical health, feeling like the experience 'put ten years on their life' and that their partner's suicide attempt marked the beginning of their own downward journey physically as well as emotionally. A large scale meta-analysis of over 300 empirical studies (a total of 18,941 participants) conducted by Segerstrom and Miller (2004) highlights the possible somatic impact from psychological stress that was also noted in the current study. Their analysis looked at a relationship between psychological stress and human immune functioning. The analysis found that chronic stressors (e.g. care-giving for a partner with dementia, or a partner becoming physically disabled) produced negative effects in nearly all aspects of the immune system. These effects were equal across all age groups and sexes. In addition, physical vulnerability as a function of age or disease also raised the likelihood of immune change during stressful times. In other words, the older the individual and the less healthy she or he is, the less able she or he is to physically withstand stress.

In the context of the present study, one middle-aged participant's physical deterioration is noteworthy, in particular due to its close proximity to her partner's suicide attempt and medical opinion that its genesis was stress related and specific to the suicide attempt. What began as relatively low-grade back pain prior to the attempt quickly developed into fibromyalgia, a chronic incurable syndrome that affects mostly women and manifests as burning pain in or around joints. It is viewed as idiopathic (without clear cause) but some studies purport that symptoms are caused by the body reacting to intense psychological stress (Irish Health, 2021).

Summary

All participants in this study experienced their partner's attempted suicide as traumatic. In addition, a significant proportion of participants were confronted with reactivation of childhood trauma that they believe was triggered by their partner's suicide attempt. These experiences had the effect of transforming them in 'being' because at once nothing was ever the same again and their traumatic exposure became a lens through which they were experiencing the world. Transformation for participants also manifested in confronting this hitherto unresolved childhood trauma and working through it in various ways in an attempt to integrate it in some way. Some participants were more successful at this than others. Some evidence was also gleaned from the current study that the significant psychological stress caused by the suicide attempt precipitated the adverse transformation of the body manifesting in chronic illness for a number of participants.

Transformation through ambiguous loss

The experience of grief and loss as a repercussion of a suicide attempt is one that needs to be validated for relatives and significant others (Popadiuk, 2005). There are many ways to conceptualize grief but many theories of grief are now considerably outdated as they emphasized a linear model of grieving with an end goal of 'letting go' of the deceased. New models of grief view loss as a complex and individual process that is non-linear in nature.

Many authors (Doka, 2002; Attig, 2004; Worden, 2009) describe the experience of 'disenfranchised grief' in the context of completed suicide that is, a loss that is viewed as being socially unspeakable. With 'completed suicide' there is clarity in the permanency of the death. However, with regard to the suicide attempt of a loved one, death has not occurred but the grief of a 'significant other' is disenfranchized *and* the nature of the loss ambiguous.

> Unlike death, an ambiguous loss may never allow people to achieve the detachment that is necessary for normal closure. Just as ambiguity complicates loss, it complicates the mourning process. People can't start grieving because the situation is indeterminate. It feels like a loss but it is not really one. (Boss, 1999, p. 10)

Ambiguous loss can be conceptualized as a relational disorder that is unclear and traumatic. It is externally caused rather than through individual pathology, and is incredibly difficult to process (Boss, 2010; Dahl and Boss, 2020). With ambiguous loss the individual is still here, but not fully here; therefore, there is neither an official notice of the loss nor a ritual to mark it. Ordinarily, communities support families in resolving loss through mourning, funeral and other rituals but, for losses that are not obvious no validation from the community is usually forthcoming. Two main types of ambiguous loss have been conceptualized (Boss, 2010; Dahl and Boss, 2020).

1. Physical absence with psychological presence: a

significant other is missing physically but kept psychologically present. This can manifest as a result of a loved one being lost, kidnapped, or more familiarly through adoption, separation/divorce, or immigration.

2. Physical presence with psychological absence: a significant other is present physically but for whatever reason missing psychologically. This can be manifested through illnesses such as Alzheimer's disease and other dementias (Boss, 2010), as well as the result of acquired brain injury (Landau and Hissett, 2008), heart attack, stroke, coma, depression (O'Brien, 2007), addiction, obsessive–compulsive behaviours, or fixation with work (Boss, 2010).

A psychotherapist whose partner experienced an acquired brain injury highlights the intensity of her ambiguity, an experience that may resonate for partners of attempted suicide:

How is it possible to lose half a person? Half is dead, half remains alive ... the uncanny story violates the observer's trust in reality. Life may then deceive by promising substance and delivering ghosts. The doppelganger sits at the dinner table. (Feilgeson, 1993, p. 335)

Boss (1999; 2016) first identified the phenomenon of ambiguous loss in 1974 through research with the families of pilots missing in action (MIA) in Vietnam and Cambodia. Interviews with 47 families throughout California, Hawaii, and Europe found that increased conflict and general dysfunction existed in those families where the wife of the

MIA pilot invested in keeping him 'psychologically' present despite his 'physical' absence. Thus, wives who consistently communicated to children in a way that implied the imminent return of their father, 'wait until your father gets home!', displayed more psychological and emotional disturbance, as did their children. A later study by Boss, Pearce-McCall, and Greenberg (1987) surveyed 140 parents whose adolescent children had recently left home and found that there was a positive correlation between the parents' perception of their absent adolescent as being still 'present' and the level of parental distress. More specifically, greater parental anxiety, depression, sleep disruption, negativity and illness, particularly among fathers, was associated with having recurrent thoughts about their welfare, difficulty accepting that their children had grown up, and yearning for their return home. Later research developed the study of 'psychological' absence of a family member. The families of 70 individuals with Alzheimer's were assessed for depressive symptomatology and again three years later. Boss (1999) found that the best predictor of depression was not the severity of the patient's illness but rather the caregiver's perception of whether the patient was 'present' or 'absent' within the family.

The literature to date, however, has not recognized the phenomenon that is the psychological absence arising from the suicide attempt of a loved one and its possible resulting ambiguous loss for partners. Partners of individuals who have attempted suicide may have to cope with both the intentional nature of the attempter's behaviour, that is, knowing their partner intended to die through their own volition, and also the ambiguity surrounding their continued presence/absence.

Since ambiguous loss entails a loved one being either psychologically present but *physically* absent or physically present but *psychologically* absent, the individual can be deemed 'here' but 'not here' to some degree. Partners or other family members can experience their grief as 'frozen' in time and as a consequence forces life to be put on hold (Boss, 2010).The potentially debilitating, intrusive, pervasive nature of ambiguous loss establishes it as a trauma:

> … ambiguous loss is traumatic because it is painful, immobilizing, and incomprehensible so that coping is blocked. It is akin to the trauma that causes post-traumatic stress disorder (PTSD) in that it is a painful experience far beyond normal human expectations. But unlike PTSD, it remains in the present; that is, the traumatizing experience (the ambiguity) often continues for years, a lifetime, or even across generations… (Boss, 2010, p. 139)

Boss (2010) conceptualizes ambiguous loss as the most complicated type of loss because it is traumatic in nature, its cause is external and so out of the sufferer's control, and because there is no closure, which is generally the ultimate goal of grief therapy. In essence, there is *no* resolution of grief (Boss, 1999; 2010; 2020). Participants in this study experienced ambiguous loss that was adversely transformative for them as the experience of their partner's attempted suicide profoundly impacted their view of their family unit and roles within it, their partner, their relationship and their view of themselves within that relationship. Participants' perception of the suicide attempt as a 'show stopper' and 'monumental' reflects how influential the experience was for them and the degree to which it transformed their everyday lives. Participants were 'transformed' in *being* as a result of their ambiguous loss and *functioning* as a result of having to re-evaluate the 'psychological family' (see 'Boundary ambiguity', below).

Boss (2007; 2016) actively encourages the continued application of ambiguous loss theory to heretofore unstudied populations and/or situations. Her research to date has highlighted the prevalence of ambiguous loss in both common situations (e.g. adoption, divorce, children leaving home, and obsession with work, internet, computer games) and catastrophic or unexpected situations such as missing persons, incarceration, dementias, addictions, chronic mental illness, depression, traumatic brain injury, and coma (Boss, 2004). The trauma of all of the aforementioned ambiguous losses are felt:

> ...when there is a sudden change from the ordinary dependable way things are in everyday life to the extraordinary and bizarre distortions that occur when a known person is profoundly altered. (Feilgeson, 1993, p. 332)

At a conference on 'supporting individuals and families in transition' in 2011 Pauline Boss communicated that she could see great value in pursuing research into the interrelationship of the experience of attempted suicide, ambiguous loss and boundary ambiguity for partners (personal communication, Webster University Conference: *Building Bridges: Supporting Individuals and Families in Transition*, 19–21 October 2011, Geneva).

Participants in the current study experienced loss that was devastating to them in the wake of their partner's suicide attempt. For some the loss came with a realization that their partner had made preparations to die some time before the suicide attempt, all the while living a seemingly 'normal' life with them and their children. Participants now knew that their partners had turned *away* from them rather than towards them in their darkest hour. This challenged their assumptions about the quality of their relationship and about the identity of the person they fell in love with.

The exposure to a loved one's suicide attempt left participants in the current study experiencing ambiguous loss of the kind that had the continued physical presence of their partner but his or her *psychological absence*. Participants described their partner as having emotionally and cognitively 'checked out' following their suicide attempt. Some described their partner as becoming a 'zombie' which was related to their sense of shame, their avoidance of providing an explanation for their suicide attempt, their consumption of heavy psychotropic medication or a combination of these. Some participants found that their partner was reluctant to engage with them after the attempt and there was a reluctance to answer questions about the 'whys?' of their suicide attempt, with responses becoming more and more measured over time. Participants experienced a 'psychological' distancing instigated by their partners which resulted in a bizarre situation of recognizing their partner physically but experiencing them as someone they knew less and less. This is reminiscent of the type of ambiguous loss experienced by individuals whose partners are physically present but become less recognizable to them as a result of dementia, addiction, depression, and chronic mental illness.

Boundary ambiguity

When Pauline Boss (1999) first identified the phenomenon of ambiguous loss in 1974/1975 through research with the families of pilots missing in action (that is, physical absence with psychological presence) she also identified that:

> ... neither physical presence nor physical absence tells the whole story of who is in and who is out of people's lives, because there is also a psychological family. (Boss, 1999, pp. 13–14)

The 'psychological family' (Boss, 2018) refers to the absence or presence of family members being a *psychological* as well as a physical concept. Boss (2006) highlights the significance of *perception* here in that how family members perceive ambiguous loss is connected to their perception of the degree of 'boundary ambiguity' within it.

With its origins in family stress theory, the concept of

boundary ambiguity was first conceptualized in the 1970s and refers to 'a state when family members are uncertain in their *perception* of who is in or out of the family or who is performing what *roles* and *tasks* within the family system' (Boss, 1987, p. 709). From a family systems point of view then, a lack of certainty about the physical and psychological presence or absence of a family member can become a significant stressor. This stressor can have a considerable impact with higher levels of ambiguity creating greater levels of helplessness and dysfunction, in particular conflict and depression. Some normal life-span family boundary changes can occur such as the addition of a child or employment-related absences. Rapoport (1963), in her research on normative family stress and boundaries, described these critical transition points as 'points-of-no-return'. Carroll, Olson and Buckmiller (2007) in their thirty-year review of theory, research, and measurement of boundary ambiguity found that it has been comprehensively researched across eleven domains including: divorce, missing-in-action, stepfamilies, clergy families, illness and care giving, and death. However, no prior research appears to have considered the boundary ambiguity for partners attached to the 'half-death' that occurs after an attempted suicide. The findings of the current study would suggest that the experience of their partner's attempt was transformational for participants in that it signposted a 'point-of-no-return' in how they perceived the organization of the family system.

Ordinarily there is either an overt or a covert perception among family members of who is in or out of the family

(Boss, Greenberg and Pearce-McCall, 1990; Dahl and Boss, 2020). Participants in the current study experienced a high degree of boundary ambiguity following their partner's suicide attempt due to their perception of their partner being no longer emotionally available to the system. Participants struggled with interpreting their new reality of the family and so this became a source of ambiguity. Some participants became ambiguous about where they located *themselves* within the context of the family system, experiencing a desire to withdraw or opt out of the system, which compounded an already complex situation. Ironically, for some participants this resulted in psychologically excluding the suicide attempter despite his or her physical presence. They described their 'reflex to share' with their partner having all but disappeared. Others talked about no longer consulting their partner or asking advice about important life matters that they would almost certainly have approached them about heretofore. This phenomenon has also been reported in families with a terminally ill or an alcoholic family member (Boss *et al.*, 1990).

There are a number of theoretical propositions from the boundary ambiguity and theory development project developed by Boss in the period 1975–1988 (Boss *et al.*, 1990) that may serve to shed more light on the possible implications of boundary ambiguity for participants in this study such as the greater the boundary ambiguity, the greater the stress with individual and family dysfunction; if a high level of boundary ambiguity remains for an extended period, the system can become stressed and ultimately dysfunctional; and the culture within which the family exists will influence the family's perception of an event. Individual differences occurred for participants in this study regarding the degree to which each was able to tolerate and assimilate information about the loss, so as to begin a process of structural reorganization (Boss 1980; Boss et al., 1990; Dahl and Boss, 2020). For some participants while the journey was at times harrowing they managed to cognitively and interpersonally restructure the 'meaning of the event of the loss' (Boss et al., 1990, p. 5) in order to regain clarity around the boundaries of the family system and return to a state of homeostasis:

> Stress continues in any family until membership can be clarified and the system reorganized regarding (a) who performs what roles and tasks, and (b) how family members perceive the absent member. (Boss, 1980, p. 21)

For some participants 'countering the torment' associated with boundary ambiguity involved keeping the lines of communication open with their spouse, identifying a cause for the attempt that they could live with, and attempting to extrapolate some meaning from the event. Another strategy was to ensure that their spouse took a more active role within the family system, for example, encouraging active participation with the children, carrying out apparently menial tasks like emptying the dishwasher or putting washing out, and ensuring she or he maintained personal responsibility for their own basic needs (food, personal hygiene) and for seeking out professional support in the community. None of these were achieved soon after the suicide attempt, but over time as participants learned to adjust to the ambiguity associated with the loss and the boundaries within the system.

For other participants their ability to find a meaning for the psychological absence of their partner that they could live with was not as achievable. Some participants described the dynamic changing from living together to living side by side, or having lost respect for their partner and their ability to trust, which they felt was fundamental to a functional relationship. Recall the participant who knew almost instantaneously following her husband's attempt that she could not resolve this in order to sustain the relationship, and another participant who repeated the mantra to himself 'get her better and then you can leave':

> Non-resolution of boundary ambiguity holds the family at a higher stress level by blocking the regenerative power to reorganize and develop new levels of organization. Boundaries of the system cannot be maintained, so the viability of the system is blurred. (Boss, 1980, p. 19)

These participants deeply questioned the viability of being able to maintain the system into the future. Of note here is that this seemed to occur where the suicide attempters displayed a very high degree of psychological absence. They were either unable or unmotivated to recognize and acknowledge the participant's experience, which appeared to adversely influence the participant's ability to resolve the boundary ambiguity. At the time of interview, some participants found it challenging to see their marriage intact into the future. From their point of view the attachment in the relationship had been irrevocably damaged.

This is the first known study of its kind to propose a link between ambiguous loss and the experience of individuals following a partner's suicide attempt. It therefore, provides a valuable contribution to understanding the specific needs of this previously forgotten population.

Transformation through attachment injury

Attachment theory has become one of the most well-known and influential theories spanning early childhood development to adult relationships. Bowlby (1988) highlighted our capacity to form powerful affectional bonds with significant people in our lives and the positive influences these bonds have on how we experience the world. A 'secure' attachment bond within a couple relationship emphasizes reciprocity in which both partners experience comfort, closeness and security. It stands to reason, therefore, that a violation of this affectional bond can have far-reaching consequences for both the injured party and by extension the relationship itself. Johnson, Makinen and Millikin (2001) first articulated these 'negative attachment-related events' (p.145) as 'attachment injuries' which are injuries that usually manifest in the form of betrayals and abandonment. An attachment injury is, therefore, perpetrated:

...when one partner violates the expectation that the other will offer comfort and caring in times of danger or distress. This incident becomes a clinically recurring theme and creates an impasse that blocks relationship repair. (Johnson *et al.*, 2001, p. 145)

The construct of attachment injury first came to light during emotionally focused couples therapy. Therapists witnessed couples maintaining distress despite successfully negotiating an impasse in the relationship (Johnson, 1996). This appeared to be connected with couples getting stuck in a 'blame/defend' cycle as a result of an unresolved specific incident in which one partner experienced betrayal by the other.

Feeney (2005), in her studies of hurt feelings in couple relationships, explored the role of attachment and perception of personal injury. 'Personal injury' was defined as 'damage to the victim's view of self as worthy of love and/or to core beliefs about the availability and trustworthiness of others' (Feeney, 2005, p. 256). This research postulated that 'hurt' is an emotional response to 'relationship transgressions' that induce a sense of personal injury and a low relational evaluation. Leary (2001) concurs with placing perception of relationship devaluation as a central feature of hurtful events and describes it as the perception that the 'offender' views the relationship as less significant or close than the other partner would prefer. Vangelisti (2001) has also highlighted the importance of a partner's *appraisal* of the event as intentionally hurtful or not. Various types of hurtful events have been suggested specifically in the context of romantic relationships (Feeney, 2004):

1. active disassociation (rejection, abandonment, withdrawing feelings of love)
2. passive disassociation (eliminating partner from activities or ignoring partner)
3. criticism (subtle or overt belittling)
4. sexual infidelity
5. deception (lying to, misleading, betraying confidence).

The suicide attempt of a spouse was appraised by participants variously as a form of disassociation (both active and passive) and as a form of deception. A number of participants in the current study articulated their perception of having been betrayed by their partner as a result of his or her suicide attempt. They described a total violation in trust and a sense of abandonment for both themselves and their children, which for them exacerbated the injury. The experience was transformational for participants in that it profoundly altered how they saw their world, themselves, and their relationship. Participants were forced to confront the illusion of knowing their partners *inside out* and that they would consistently create a 'safe haven' for comfort and protection (Bowlby, 1969).

Two factors seemed to mediate the extent of the injury for participants. First was the participant's perception of the degree to which their partner (the suicide attempter) acknowledged their hurt and made concerted efforts to reassure and repair the relationship. Second was the participant's willingness or ability to accept this reassurance from their partner:

> Much depends on how the injured partner interprets the event in question and how the other spouse responds to expressions of hurt by the injured party. When this spouse discounts, denies, or dismisses the injury, this prevents the processing of the event in the relationship and compounds the injury. (Johnson *et al.*, 2001, p. 149)

This is particularly relevant in the context of the current study where, in the eyes of some participants, the suicide attempter was very much absorbed in their own experience to the extent that they did not recognize, nor adequately respond to, their partner's hurt. For some participants their attachment injury came to the fore very shortly after becoming cognisant of their partner's attempt – some of the suicide attempters asked after their mothers and other family-of-origin members immediately on regaining consciousness rather than desiring to see their own spouse. This left participants dazed, hurt and confused about the 'security' of their bond with their partner and questioning the profound interdependence that is supposedly part and parcel of a healthy, loving relationship.

A transformational aspect of this experience may have occurred in the context of participants' 'internal working models' of self (lovable vs unlovable) and others (responsive/accessible vs unresponsive/inaccessible) that significantly influence how they relate to other adults (Bowlby, 1979). Their partner's suicide attempt may have challenged their internal working model of self as 'lovable'. The same might apply to their internal working model of 'other'.

Some of the participants in the current study emphasized their perception of the suicide attempt as a betrayal and that their partner was abandoning both them and their children. Similar feelings have been found to surface as defining moments during times such as physical threat or uncertainty (for example, illness), loss (for example, miscarriage), or transitions (for example, retirement). However, what seems to be paramount across all of these events is the impact it has on the attachment as evaluated by the 'injured' partner, rather than on the specific content of each event. Some experienced the betrayal as a trauma. In fact Atkinson (1997) considers attachment theory itself as a 'theory of trauma' due to its potentially injurious impact on people given the right circumstances. 'Trauma' comes from the Latin word 'to wound' which resonates with the shattering of one's assumptive world outlined earlier. It also serves to highlight what might be called the 'shadow side' of the partner's experience, that is, the side of their experience that constitutes feelings of hurt and betrayal that is not recognized or sanctioned by society. Johnson *et al.,* (2001) describe the onset of 'existential vulnerability' with the potential for symptoms reminiscent of PTSD:

> Memories and emotions connected to the event linger and manifest themselves in the form of dreams, flashbacks, and intrusive memories. Much energy may be spent in ruminating about every minute detail of

the event and the reasons why it occurred. Offending partners may apologize for their transgressions, but injured partners cannot let the matter go. These events are pivotal moments in the ongoing definition of the relationship that constantly come up and color present realities. (Johnson *et al.*, 2001, p. 150)

For some other participants in the current study, however, part of their trauma was related to their perception that *they* had inflicted an attachment injury on their *partner*. Participants in this light saw themselves as having perpetrated the 'crime' of 'not seeing it coming' and not being adequately attentive to their spouse who they knew at some level was stressed or busy or distracted in some way. The bottom line for these participants was that they felt they had not responded adequately to their partner's needs and consequently violated the sanctity of the secure emotional bond by failing to encourage 'proximity seeking' behaviour, failing to create a 'secure base', failing to create a 'safe haven', and failing to resist separation (Bowlby, 1969). This manifested for these participants as self-blame and ultimately had the effect of increasing their tendency to offer reassurance to both their partners and significant others. Some participants in fact, perceived having experienced a combination of the two whereby, they had, at once been both victim to an attachment injury through their spouse's attempt, as well as inflicting an attachment injury by not responding to the needs of their spouse pre- and post-suicide attempt.

Although some participants have continued to live with the deleterious effects of their partner's suicide attempt both for themselves and for their romantic relationship, others significantly have been able to experience what can only be described as 'positive transformation' across many domains of their life *in spite of* their traumatic stress.

Positive transformation: post-traumatic growth

A number of authors have championed the notion of positive psychological transformation as a result of experiencing a very stressful or traumatic event. Tedeschi, Calhoun, Morrell and Johnson first introduced the term 'transformation of trauma' in a paper presented in 1984 on grief and psychological development (Tedeschi and Calhoun 2004). Aldwin (1994) introduced the concept of 'transformational coping' in the context of development through stress. Grof (2000) noted that 'spiritual emergencies', usually as a result of traumatic experiences, had the capacity to bring about 'spiritual emergence' that encompassed permanent positive changes for the individual. Joseph and Linley (2005) have developed 'organismic valuing theory' suggesting that the individual has an innate drive to always move towards growth. Taylor (2012) has described 'suffering-induced transformational experiences' or SITEs in his research on positive psychological transformation after episodes of intense turmoil. Bray (2013) discusses the potential for transformation in the aftermath of bereavement. The research conducted by Calhoun and Tedeschi is the most comprehensive of its kind and will, therefore, be the focus for this section on positive transformation.

While they would submit that the idea of positive change emanating from suffering has an ancient history, Calhoun and Tedeschi have arguably been the most influential in developing this construct empirically, particularly from the 1990s when they first coined the term *post-traumatic growth* (PTG):

Posttraumatic growth describes the experience of individuals whose development, at least in some areas, has surpassed what was present before the struggle with crises occurred. The individual has not only survived, but has experienced changes that are viewed as important, and that go beyond what was the previous status quo. Posttraumatic growth is not simply a return to baseline – it is an experience of improvement that for some persons is deeply profound. (Tedeschi and Calhoun, 2004, p.4)

Zautra, Hall and Murray (2010) have described the concept of resilience whereby individuals with particular personality traits or coping mechanisms have greater potential to sustain themselves through a life crisis and recover to pre-trauma baseline levels of functioning. Tedeschi and Calhoun (2004), however, stress that post-traumatic growth is much more than just resilience or similar concepts such as hardiness or optimism, creating a change in people that:

... goes beyond an ability to resist and not be damaged by highly stressful circumstances; it involves a movement beyond pretrauma levels of adaptation. Posttraumatic growth, then, has the quality of transformation ... (Tedeschi and Calhoun, 2004, p.4)

They make an important observation in that growth does not occur as a *direct* result of a trauma itself, but instead is positively correlated with the extent to which a person is able to make sense of their new reality. There are a large number of life crises that have prompted post-traumatic growth for people including bereavement, arthritis, HIV infection, cancer, heart attack, coping with ill children, house fires, sexual assault, combat, being a refugee and being taken hostage (Tedeschi and Calhoun, 2004). The trauma of a partner's suicide attempt can now be added to this catalogue of events because, for most of the participants in the current study, their traumatic journey also entailed growth in fundamental ways. Tedeschi and Calhoun (2004) have developed five domains from their research in which people tend to experience growth following a trauma:

1. relating to others (more meaningful and compassionate relationships)
2. new possibilities (grasping opportunities, different roles, new relationships)
3. personal strength (feeling psychologically and emotionally stronger)
4. spiritual change (greater spiritual connection; developing, renewed or increasing faith)
5. appreciation of life (increased gratitude and enjoyment of simple aspects of life).

Participants in this study provided powerful descriptions of how they had experienced positive transformation and growth as a result of struggling through their partner's attempt. They described 'feeling blessed' and that they 'wouldn't change it [what happened to them] for the world'. Some also experienced a change in priorities, for example, investing more in their relationship through more regular communication and nights away. Some described the aftermath of their partner's suicide attempt as a time for finding their own voice, for developing more freedom, autonomy, and independence. Others described becoming a better listener and more empathic, becoming a better person, feeling a greater bond with their partner, and not fearing death the way they had prior to their trauma. All of these elements were completely unanticipated by the participants in the time just following their partner's attempt and only came to the fore during their working through the 'loss' associated with the attempt and attempting to make sense of it in a way they could live with. Tedeschi and Calhoun (2004) note that individuals do not purposely set out to create positive transformation in any particular way but that it is experienced in the midst of them attempting to 'adapt to highly negative sets of circumstances that can engender high levels of psychological distress' (p. 2).

Participants in the current study reported greater ease in perceiving the feelings of others; they were more grateful for the simplest of things in life reporting that 'you'd think you have nothing but yet you've everything'. Participants described a greater sense of groundedness, being less hurried in their thoughts and actions. The current study captured the transformative experience of individuals whose partner's attempted suicide, therefore, makes a valuable contribution to our knowledge of positive transformation in the wake of trauma.

Calhoun and Tedeschi (1998) have likened the process of growth experienced by individuals following a trauma to the experience of an earthquake and its aftermath. They describe the trauma as a psychologically 'seismic' experience that shatters or demolishes previously held schemas about how the world is supposed to operate. Our 'assumptive world' (Janoff-Bulman, 1992), mentioned earlier, becomes either severely compromised or completely obliterated:

> The 'seismic' set of circumstances severely challenges, contradicts, or may even nullify the way the individual understands why things happen, in terms of proximate causes and reasons, in terms of more abstract notions involving the general purpose and meaning of the person's existence. Such threats to the assumptive world are accompanied by significant levels of psychological distress. (Tedeschi and Calhoun, 2004, p. 4)

This metaphor resonates very much with the theme of 'the world shifting on its axis' in the current study in which participants had to find ways of adjusting to or 'countering the torment' that they were exposed to following the attempt. Countering the devastation caused by the 'seismic' event comes in the form of cognitively processing or *deliberate ruminating* over the event, so that the individual can begin the process of 'rebuilding' in a way that will potentially protect the individual from similar shocks in the future. This was borne out by some participants in the current study who suggested that they felt better equipped to cope on their own into the future in the event of their partner dying either through suicide or of natural causes:

> Cognitive rebuilding that takes into account the changed reality of one's life after the trauma produces schemas that incorporate the trauma and possible events in the future, and that are more resistant to being shattered. These results are experienced as growth. (Tedeschi and Calhoun, 2004, p. 5)

Cognitive processing of the event is usually automatic in the early aftermath which entails negative intrusive thoughts and images. For growth to occur there needs to be a strong affective component to this cognitive reprocessing, particularly if it involves the transformation of 'higher order' or fundamental goals, philosophies, or belief systems. The individual subsequently disengages from goals/schemas that have become redundant, probably over an extended period of time, thereby presenting opportunities for healthier, more deliberate rumination about the meaning and significance for individuals and their everyday lives. This fits with the experience of the participants in the current study who endured a 'desperate search for answers', particularly in the early stages. Their distress stayed with them for many months after the event, which, according to the post-traumatic growth model, needed to happen in conjunction with cognitive rebuilding so as to maximize the potential for a transformational growth experience to occur. In essence, what didn't kill them did, indeed, make them stronger but only with certain variables in play, including cognitive and affective processing.

Tedeschi and Calhoun have highlighted the potential benefit in sharing the experience with others, particularly with those who have been through something similar, in order to create new narratives. Some participants in this study did accept the support and alternative perspectives of close friends and seemed to reap rewards from this. Others, however, sought out support from no one else but reported substantial growth none the less. This adds an interesting contradiction to Tedeschi and Calhoun's model suggesting that individuals can indeed achieve transformational growth without processing the event socially. For one participant, however, she did not report growth to a transformational extent despite processing the experience socially. Both she and her medical team believe that her trauma had the effect of triggering a serious physical condition that was permanent. Thus, following the model, it may be the case that, if this participant did not experience *any* reduction in distress in the months following the trauma due to ill-health, she was less likely to experience transformational growth in the long term.

For those who experienced growth there was a paradoxical component to it insofar as there was some degree of gain in their lives out of their traumatic loss. Post-traumatic growth is postulated to have some relationship to increased wisdom for individuals as they generate new narratives for life. Although it did not *nullify* the distress of the trauma for participants in the current study, those who did experience post-traumatic growth reported an enhanced outlook on life and enhanced relationships, but not necessarily with their partners.

Summary

All participants in this study reported profound change in response to their partner's suicide attempt. The impact of the experience was that, for most, it fundamentally changed or 'transformed' them for better and for worse. Transformation occurred in 'being' for better (for example, more positive outlook on life; greater personal strength) and for worse (for example, feeling less worthy, less lovable). Transformation occurred in functioning for better (for example, taking on new roles) and for worse (for example, decline in physical health). For some, transformation happened quite abruptly, for others it was a process over time.

All participants described the experience in various ways as traumatic insofar as it instantaneously shifted their world on its axis, with nothing ever being the same again. They reported re-experiencing the event, wanting to avoid their partner's presence, negative intrusive thoughts and images, negative mood, and hypervigilance.

Participants reported a type of 'uncanny' or ambiguous loss, in which their partner was half-dead and half-alive, and in this context physically present but psychologically absent. This compounded participants' trauma in that their 'assumptive world' continued to be shattered. Participants described boundary ambiguity in that they struggled to identify if their partner was in or out of the family, or, indeed, if they themselves were in or out of the family! This was enormously stressful for participants and impacted their perception of who was performing what roles and tasks within the system.

For some participants their partner's suicide attempt was perceived as a personal injury that negatively reflected their attachment. They felt betrayed by their partner and felt that their trust had been violated. Consequently this at times impacted participant's willingness to accept reassurance from their partner. The contrary was also experienced in that some participants also felt that they were guilty of perpetrating the attachment injury for not anticipating the attachment needs of their partner.

The majority of participants in this study also experienced positive transformation in the midst of the traumatic event. 'Suffering-induced transformational experiences' or post-traumatic growth permeated cognitive, behavioural, emotional, and spiritual domains. Spiritual transformation was explicitly reported by only a small number of participants but may have been implied by others in their transformation of relating to others; of new possibilities and roles, of increased psychological and emotional strength, and in their increased appreciation of and gratitude for life.

The present study is the first of its kind to capture the in-depth lived experience of individuals whose partners have attempted suicide and survived. It captured their experience not solely from the perspective of caregiver, but, in so doing, giving participants a unique opportunity to describe the personal impact on them and their everyday lives. What permeated participant's experience across primary trauma, ambiguous loss, attachment injury, and post-traumatic growth were transformations both adverse and positive. Having a partner attempt suicide set in motion fundamental and profound change for all participants in varying ways and to varying degrees. Some aspects of their transformation were relatively short-lived whereas others appeared to hold permanent status. The personal impact on participants was traumatic on multiple levels, including the trauma of ambiguous loss, and of attachment injury. The trauma also had the effect of sowing the seeds of positive growth. All of these elements in isolation or collectively demonstrate the experience as having elicited quantum transformation (Fosha, 2006).

CHAPTER 7

Offering a new pathway of care for partners and 'others'

Introduction

The participant's extraordinary stories have made an original contri-bution to the extant literature by highlighting the transformative personal impact on partners. Studies to date have viewed partners primarily as caregivers and/or informants, with a view to developing psychotherapy's understanding of risk assessment, prevention, and recovery for those at risk of suicide. This is the first study of its kind to take an *in-depth* idiographic approach to understanding the meaning of a suicide attempt from the perspective of a partner. 'I'm not the same person I was' reflects the transformative personal impact of the experience for partners, their complex struggle with concomitant primary trauma and compassion fatigue, feeling like 'walking wounded', and desperately searching for answers. Adjusting to the trauma involved playing 'the blame game' and developing 'strategies for self-preservation', transforming their perception of self, other, and the relationship. The experience left a legacy for partners that would 'never ever go away', developing a 'routine of discomfort' as a response to adverse childhood memories, physical deterioration and changing how partners related to the suicide attempter. However, the experience, for some, also left a legacy of increased personal strength, spirituality, improved relationships and outlook on life.

This final chapter aims to draw attention to the lived experience of partners in the context of primary trauma and in so doing highlight recommendations for policy and procedure in supporting partners following an attempted suicide. Recommendations for psychotherapy practice and training will also be explored, including the significance of therapeutic goals for treating ambiguous loss, the tripartite walking in the shoes model of suicide grief as applied to attempted suicide, and betrayal as opportunity for transformation. The chapter concludes with an evaluation of theoretical transferability, and suggestions for further research in psychotherapy.

Reconfiguring 'burden of care' as primary trauma

The literature to date on the phenomenon of the personal impact of attempted suicide on partners has approached it with the sole view of the partner in the role of 'caregiver' and has conceptualized their experience in the context of 'burden of care'. The lived experience of participants in the current study revealed that it went considerably beyond the impact of caregiving. Participants experienced something that may have resembled compassion fatigue but the actual trauma of being exposed to 'the threatened death [at times violent] of a close family member' appears to have gone completely unnoticed by primary and secondary care services as documented in the available research literature, and by extension society as a whole. This is evidenced in 'Family care of Taiwanese patients who had attempted suicide: a grounded theory study' by Sun *et al.* (2008), which concluded that the priority of nursing staff was to educate family members on how to home-care patients following their discharge from hospital as well as minimizing further attempts. Although they later recognize the experience as a 'life crisis' (Sun *et al.*, 2009, p. 60) for family members, there is a presumption here that they are psychologically/ emotionally prepared and/or motivated to care for their relative following the suicide attempt.

Partners were exposed to this event first-hand, consequently their traumatic stress was *primary* in nature, causing a *downward* trajectory in their psychological and emotional health. If healthcare professionals communicate with partners solely as 'caregivers' then partners may conclude that their trauma-related feelings are both inappropriate and unjustified.

Resilience in the midst of ambiguous loss and boundary ambiguity: therapeutic interventions

It has been noted that an individual with a high degree of resiliency is more capable of navigating stress, and attaches less meaning to the trauma. Consequently s/he is less likely to develop PTSD or PTG for that matter. Resilience, therefore, is an important construct in minimizing the traumatic aftermath for individuals experiencing ambiguity associated with the attempted suicide of their partner.

Boss (2006; 2010; 2018) has proposed a number of guidelines for mental health professionals in supporting someone to develop their resiliency in the face of ambiguous loss. The participants' stories outlined in Part I serve to highlight the potential benefits of applying some of these guidelines in supporting individuals in the wake of their partner's suicide attempt. Their stories revealed that for some people gaining closure from their loss was almost impossible, given that there was no clear ending. Adapting to this 'half-death' is not straightforward and so these guidelines should be viewed as non-linear and non-prescriptive. Applying Boss's ambiguous loss theory for the first time to partners' lived experiences following an attempted suicide, I conceptualize resilience building needing to be bookended. Bookended first by what Boss describes as 'finding meaning' in the experience, one that partners can live with, and culminating at the other end with revision of attachment. In revising attachment, Boss asserts that 'there is now a categorical difference in the relationship' (2006, p. 163). Alongside finding meaning and revising attachment, Boss also proposes learning to temper mastery, normalize ambivalence, and reconstruct identity.

Finding meaning

In working phenomenologically with clients, psychotherapists can acknowledge the existence of multiple truths and recognize the client's subjective perception of an experience.

This is particularly important for individuals whose partners have attempted suicide and feel socially under pressure to perceive the event in restrictive ways (for example, 'his suicide attempt will bring you closer together').

1. A therapist first naming the problem as ambiguous loss can paradoxically enable clients to gain understanding of their experience and begin to move forward. A therapist witnessing their loss can help clients in their quest to find meaning where society does not witness the loss. Acknowledging that the only meaning for some may be that there is no meaning can be useful and can be construed as a meaning in and of itself.

2. Encouraging dialectical thinking is another important intervention that highlights both/and thinking or holding two opposing ideas simultaneously. The client acknowledges the parts of their partner that are still present and grieves for those parts that have been lost. For partners of those who have attempted suicide, this can manifest, for example, as 'He is both my husband and a stranger to me'.

3. Developing their spiritual selves or embracing their faith can improve resiliency and facilitate clients to find meaning in the midst of their ambiguity.

4. Forgiveness has also been found to facilitate resilience. Forgiving a partner's decision to hide their intention to kill themselves, or forgiving in-laws for seemingly implying that one had not shown enough 'tender-loving-care' and therefore had a hand in driving him/

her to suicide can help the search for meaning.

5. Small good works have also been found to mediate the impact of ambiguous loss and in finding meaning. Participants in the present study talked about providing a listening ear to others in a manner they had not done prior to their partner's suicide attempt or becoming an active member of a charitable mental health organization.

6. Ensuring that rituals and celebrations continue in spite of the ambiguous loss can maintain resiliency and aid in finding meaning. They may not take the same form as they used to but can provide a sense of continuity, e.g. a birthday celebration, a wedding anniversary.

7. Discovering positive attributions for the loss could significantly aid an individual's recovery. One participant I interviewed described her husband's suicide attempt as a reaction to the strain he had been putting himself under in his heroic efforts to provide for his children. Another described his wife as having always been a fighter and that her attempt didn't make her any less of a fighter. Another participant struggled with her negative attribution of his suicide attempt, which in her eyes was a complete overreaction to a minor dispute he had had with his sibling. Reframing negative attributions and finding positive ones can significantly alter an individual's perception of the experience and aid in finding meaning in it.

8. Maintaining hope is paramount to finding meaning, particularly with ambiguous loss where the future

appears very muddied. It appears likely that individuals whose partners have attempted suicide will struggle to visualize their life returning to any kind of normality or their relationship rekindling the honesty and trust that existed before the attempt. Again this underscores the importance of dialectical thinking – individuals may simultaneously experience absence/presence and anger/pity. Likewise it may be therapeutic for individuals to simultaneously hold hopelessness/hope.

9. Further guidelines in the support of those experiencing ambiguous loss in the aftermath of a partner's suicide attempt include tempering mastery, normalizing ambivalence and reconstructing identity.

Tempering mastery

Our innate need for certainty can work against us, particularly in the event of experiencing traumatic loss where ambiguity abounds. Thinking in both/and ways such as 'I am both a wife and a parent to him' is challenging for clients as it calls for them to temper their need for a sense of mastery or certainty about situations. By letting go of what is uncontrollable externally, clients can turn their attention to mastering their internal self. Tempering mastery can be facilitated by:

- helping clients to acknowledge that the world is not always fair (reminiscent of Ellis's rational–emotive behaviour therapy)
- exploring a client's worldview and core beliefs

regarding the origins of their need for mastery

- externalizing blame (that is, identifying the ambiguity as the source of their lack of mastery)
- reducing self-blame (that is, challenging clients to reframe their ideas about having had a hand in their partner's suicide attempt, for example, 'All the signs were there, I should have seen it coming')
- identifying past competencies (evidence of previous resilience), and
- championing experiences of success (that is, behavioural activation in baby steps in order to increase a sense of competence and renewed trust in the world).

Normalizing ambivalence

In the case of an individual's attempted suicide, their partner can understandably go through a rollercoaster of conflicting emotions. They may experience great joy and relief that their partner is still alive but simultaneously feel hurt and betrayed. The goal of psychotherapy here is to encourage clients to share feelings that they might assume are taboo in this context such as anger or shame. By normalizing these difficult feelings, clients can learn to manage them rather than deny them and, in so doing, increase their resilience.

Reconstructing identity

Following an individual's suicide attempt, their partner is forced to confront questions about who they are now. For example, they may ask themselves, 'Who am I now that my wife has given up on our relationship?'. Some may no longer feel like a spouse but rather a parent to their partner or merely a housemate. Established roles within the relationship may be thrown into chaos as a wife suddenly has to take on responsibility for managing faulty electrics in the house, tending to the bins and so on, much like the adjustments in roles and routines made following an actual spousal bereavement. Taking on these new roles may cause individuals to face up to their own prejudices and those of their community about what tasks are appropriate for them to undertake. Some interventions that aid identity reconstruction include:

- reducing boundary ambiguity (who is in and out of the family)
- encouraging flexibility about gender roles
- acknowledging ex-identities
- adjusting tasks regarding rituals and celebrations (for example, taking on the role of both mother and father to help a child celebrate his or her birthday during the psychological absence of the father following his suicide attempt)
- exploring the expansion of family rules regarding problem-solving (for example, a partner providing limited information to an insightful child about what has happened rather than the usual method of denying his or her awareness that something is not right).

Revising attachment

As previously mentioned, working therapeutically with ambiguous loss will never be a completely linear process as, indeed, with any grief work. That said, in terms of conceptualizing resilience building for partners, I find it helpful to bookend the process with 'finding meaning' and 'revising attachment'. The legacy of being exposed to someone close to us who has attempted suicide fundamentally transforms us as people and as a consequence transforms our attachment within the relationship.

The interviews with partners highlighted that there was often a dissonance between how society expected them to relate to the suicide attempter versus how they related in real terms. Ambivalence around provision of care thrust upon partners in the immediate aftermath of the attempt has, until now, been largely ignored. The focus in therapy, therefore, is to explore ways of continuing to relate to the suicide attempter while simultaneously sitting with the discomfort of a multitude of uncertainty and confusion – unanswered questions; ambivalent feelings oscillating between pity, compassion, anger, and betrayal; boundary ambiguity; and a partner who is less available than ever before. Boss (2006) champions the therapeutic relationship as a significant driver in processing the trauma of ambiguous loss. The experience of positive transference is viewed as paramount within the context of individual psychotherapy, whereas increasing trust is of central importance within the context of couples therapy. Although cognitive–behavioural approaches will look to realign distorted thinking and encourage increased social engagement and activity, Boss emphasizes psychodynamic, relational and narrative psychotherapeutic approaches to aid the client in developing various alternative narratives in order to assimilate the event of the suicide attempt. This encompasses the therapist being reflexive about their own cultural beliefs and being sensitive to the cultural background of the client. It also entails encouraging open expression of feelings normally not socially sanctioned, including moving from despair to protest (Boss, 2006) as well as, in the context of partners, possible feelings of hurt, betrayal, and relationship injury. The process of revising attachment will ideally be undertaken through both individual psychotherapy and couple therapy, where the outcome will encompass either post-traumatic growth within the relationship, a deterioration or impasse within the relationship, or a termination of the love relationship involving separation.

Transformative learning and the tripartite walking in the shoes model of suicide grief as applied to *attempted* suicide

Tranformative learning first conceptualized by Mezirow (1990) has its origins in andragogy (adult learning theory). In this context it is thought that transformation can occur in response to a 'disorienting dilemma', that is, a challenge to one's world view or frame of reference. Beyond adult education, however, transformative learning has been shown to be applicable to disorienting dilemmas triggered by a 'life

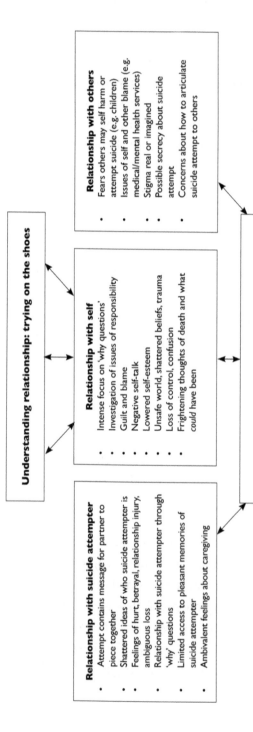

Understanding relationship: trying on the shoes

Relationship with others
- Fears others may self harm or attempt suicide (e.g. children)
- Issues of self and other blame (e.g. medical/mental health services)
- Stigma real or imagined
- Possible secrecy about suicide attempt
- Concerns about how to articulate suicide attempt to others

Relationship with self
- Intense focus on 'why questions'
- Investigation of issues of responsibility
- Guilt and blame
- Negative self-talk
- Lowered self-esteem
- Unsafe world, shattered beliefs, trauma
- Loss of control, confusion
- Frightening thoughts of death and what could have been

Relationship with suicide attempter
- Attempt contains message for partner to piece together
- Shattered ideas of who suicide attempter is
- Feelings of hurt, betrayal, relationship injury, ambiguous loss
- Relationship with suicide attempter through 'why' questions
- Limited access to pleasant memories of suicide attempter
- Ambivalent feelings about caregiving

Reconstructing relationship: walking in the shoes

Relationship with others
- Prioritizing concerns for ongoing safety of suicide attempter
- Unable to voice own trauma, relationship injury, and grief
- Ongoing fear for safety of others (e.g. children)
- Withdrawn socially

Relationship with self
- Intense inward focus on pain of suicide attempter's life
- Meaning-making difficulties
- Re-enactment of time leading up to suicide attempt and personal narrative of event by suicide attempter him or herself
- Questioning everything, possibly including value of living
- Differentiation from the behaviour associated with the suicide attempt

Relationship with suicide attempter
- Take on his or her mindset
- Withdrawn
- Trying to imagine emotional and physical turmoil in their life up to, and during, the suicide attempt, either separate or co-constructed with suicide attempter
- Inability to make meaning of self-volition of suicide attempt at sufficient emotional level
- Difficulty accepting that suicide attempter would knowingly inflict pain on the family

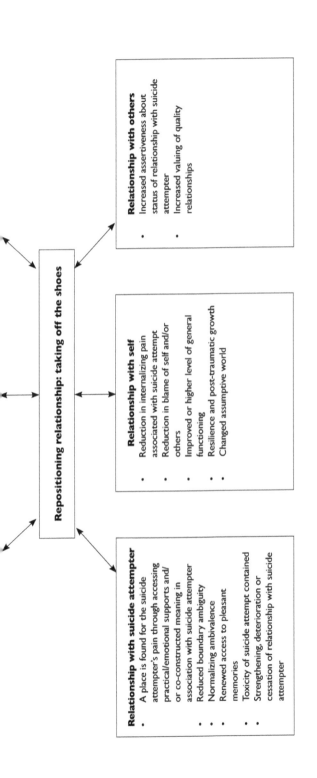

Figure 2 *The tripartite walking in the shoes model of attempted suicide grief, adapted from the tripartite walking in the shoes model of suicide grief (Neimeyer and Sands, 2017)*

crisis' such as illness, unemployment and bereavement. The resulting disorienting dilemma triggers critical reflection which 'enables us to correct distortions in our beliefs' (Mezirow, 1990, p. 1). Critical reflection ultimately facilitates meaning-making out of a 'chaotic situation that was not understandable from within existing meaning frameworks' (Mälkki, 2012, p. 207). The challenge for an individual in chaos is to transform their meaning perspective in the midst of essentially being in a 'vacuum of meanings', where 'one is neither able to imagine one's life ahead as based on one's previous experiences nor able to have coherent anticipations of the future' (Mälkki, 2012, p. 209). More recent empirical investigations applying the paradigm of transformative learning, have explored the emotional dimension of transformation as well as the social construction of meaning perspectives (Taylor, 2007). These include life crises such as elder bereavement (Moon, 2011), involuntary childlessness (Mälkki, 2012) and suicide bereavement (Sands and Tennant, 2010).

Sands and Tennant's study (2010) aimed to understand the various aspects associated with the 'healing and meaning-making' processes of those bereaved by suicide. A group case study method of data collection was employed capturing several forms of data during suicide bereavement group workshops (sixteen male and female participants). Three core themes were identified that facilitated meaning-making and were conceptualized through a relational lens. The first theme, 'intentionality', represents the bereaved individual's emotional attempt to understand why their deceased relative chose to take their own life, involving a process of 'trying on the shoes' of the deceased. The second theme, 'walking in the shoes', represents an effort to reconstruct the death scene, the deceased's life prior to the suicide and the meaning the suicide has for the bereaved in the context of the relationship. The final theme, 'taking off the shoes', represents the bereaved individual's ability to move beyond their relative's decision to die, thereby creating new meaning and integrating the death. Sands and Tennant (2010) conclude that the process of meaning-making experienced by those bereaved by suicide reflected the phases of transformative learning namely:

A disorienting dilemma; a self examination; with feelings of fear, anger, guilt, or shame; a sharing of experiences with others; the exploration of new roles; and a reintegration of a new perspective in one's life. (Sands and Tennant, 2010, p.114)

The significance of the emotional dimension within transformative learning has been highlighted by Sands and Tennant. In essence, the more open one is to working through emotions, both positive and negative, the more open to reflection, and thereby transformation, one becomes. In addition, the significance of the social dimension within transformative learning has been noted by both Sands and Tennant (2010) and Mälkki (2012), who describes a 'second-wave' trigger for reflection in which social engagement during a disorienting dilemma can create further disorienting dilemmas as a result of new disagreements with significant others that come to the surface.

Sands and Tennant's study highlights the applicability of Mezirow's transformative learning theory to those bereaved through suicide and the role of meaning-making in the context of relationship with the self, the deceased and significant others. Taking the position that the study is one within a 'highly emotionally charged context' (Sands and Tennant, 2010, p. 100), the researchers view the transformative learning experience as one during which individuals experience profound change in 'being'. In the context of the my own study, Sun *et al.* (2009) have identified a suicide attempt as a 'life crisis' for family members. Therefore, partners may experience a 'disorienting dilemma' in response to this highly emotional event, with possible 'second-wave' dilemmas experienced on the basis of social interaction. This may have important implications for supporting this vulnerable group psychotherapeutically in their meaning-making process and ultimately in 'being'.

The personal impact on participants following the attempted suicide of their loved one, as seen through their personal accounts in Part 1 of this book, was found to be very similar to the impact described by individuals in Sands and Tennant's (2010) study following their bereavement through an actual suicide. Sands' (2009) developed the 'tripartite' model of suicide grief on the basis of the aforementioned study, now known as the 'Tripartite Walking in the Shoes Model' (Neimeyer and Sands, 2017; McGann, Sands, and Gutin, in press). An adapted version of this model may prove beneficial for psychotherapists and other professionals, such as community mental health nurses, in facilitating partners coming to terms with the suicide attempt. As Boss (2006;

2010) has outlined in the treatment of ambiguous loss, Sands (2009) has also highlighted the importance of the 'meaning-making' journey that those bereaved by suicide take.

An adapted version of the tripartite walking in the shoes model as applied to attempted suicide (Figure 2) could potentially facilitate a partner in making sense of their loved one's suicide attempt and in doing so adapting to a 'new normal' in which this experience is integrated into the relationship with the self, the suicide attempter, and others. The reader should note that there are some subtle but significant differences between the two models. The suggested adapted model, as applied to attempted suicide, should be viewed as a tentative first step in setting the foundation for developing a deeper understanding of the experience of partners and, thereby, could be subject to review following further research. The tripartite walking in the shoes model offers three phases of grief that are by no means linear in nature. The bi-directional arrows highlight the back and forth nature of this complicated process as partners strive to negotiate the various relational aspects involved.

In exploring the first phase of 'intentionality', partners could be encouraged to 'try on the shoes' of the suicide attempter and make some kind of sense of their intention towards death. It heavily involves, 'Why?' questions, such as 'Why didn't she come and talk to me?'; questions about level of intent, such as 'To what extent did he really want to die?'; and questions casting doubt upon the quality of their relationship, such as 'Did she think about me at any point leading up to her suicide attempt?'.

The second phase, involving 'reconstruction' of the death story, would, in the adapted version, encourage partners to 'walk in their shoes' with the aim of trying to understand the mindset of the individual who made the attempt and what psychological and emotional pain they were going through that prompted such an extreme behaviour. Unlike the original model, the individual who attempted suicide is still alive but this does not necessarily guarantee that answers will be forthcoming or, indeed, that a partner will always feel motivated to engage in a dialogue with a view to empathizing with their experience. A significant challenge for partners working through this phase of the model would be to differentiate themselves in that they want to live while acknowledging that the suicide attempter wanted to die and perhaps still wants to die.

The third and final phase of the model highlights 'repositioning' of the relationship or 'taking off the shoes', denoting the re-engagement in relationship with the self, and others, but also an ongoing relationship with their partner (rather than with the deceased as in the original model). Akin to 'revising attachment' previously highlighted in the context of ambiguous loss, 'repositioning' may also culminate in the termination of the love relationship within the couple and them going their separate ways.

Sand's tripartite walking in the shoes model may be a useful aid in individual psychotherapy for partners working through grief associated with an attempted suicide. However, it may also prove useful in a couple-therapy context where the couple negotiate 'repositioning' of the relationship. The following section offers a conceptualization of hurt and loss associated with a suicide attempt as an opportunity to transform the relationship.

Attachment injury as opportunity for transformation

The 'father of suicidology', Shneidman, contended that most suicidal acts are essentially dyadic events, that is, there are ramifications not only for the suicide attempter but, for the 'significant other' (Leenaars, 2010). The finding in this study that participants perceived a sense of betrayal, abandonment, and violation of trust in response to their partner's attempted suicide pointed to the literature on attachment injury as a result of 'relationship transgressions'. This finding indicates that the potential consequences of a suicide attempt within the couple context are far-reaching and that interventions focusing on minimizing risk regarding further suicide attempts and advising partners within the care-giving context tell only half the story. Participants believed that the suicide attempt reflected a low opinion of the relationship on the part of the suicide attempter, and consequently some either left the relationship or thought about leaving. Warren, Morgan, Williams and Mansfield (2008) offer a three-stage psychotherapeutic model aimed at couples following an affair which may prove useful in exploring betrayal within the context of a suicide attempt. The model is creative and metaphor-based, and therefore chosen to potentially facilitate both parties visualizing moving beyond the attempted suicide with the relationship intact. It is premised on a traditional Buddhist tale about how we can choose to manage a poisoned tree in one of three ways: cutting the tree down as it is viewed as both no longer useful and no longer viable; building a wall around the tree in recognition of its history but simultaneously recognizing it as a threat to ourselves and others; or taking a deeper perspective and seeing the potentially healing properties the poison has to offer when combined with other ingredients. It is suggested that infidelity can be reframed as an 'opportunity for transformation':

> Using a metaphor such as the poisoned tree can help couples distance themselves from the emotional chaos, even if only slightly, and find a new perspective as well as a path for potential healing. (Warren *et al.*, 2008, p. 351)

Stage one, entitled 'do not cut down the tree', encourages a shifting of perspective for the betrayed partner from blame, a desire for retribution and/or separation, and any other behaviours that could be construed as reactivity. Instead the couple is urged to slow the process down and view it as an opportunity for deeper insight and growth. The key question at this stage is 'If the infidelity could speak, what would it say?' (Warren *et al.*, 2008, p.353).

Stage two, 'steps to protecting the tree from further harm', explores how each partner can protect the other partner and the relationship from encountering further harm. The couple are encouraged to construe the *poison* as problematic rather than the tree itself. The source of the poison, therefore, is explored, such as, unhealthy family of origin patterns of relating; a partner's view of self, other, and the world; and ways in which they cope with adversity. Considering the metaphor of the poisoned tree, these early patterns represent the soil in which the tree is planted and so may require considerable attention in order to not only preserve the tree but also enhance its well-being. Forgiveness (Dupree *et al.*, 2007) is considered a significant aspect of this stage of the model where apologies from both parties can be forthcoming due to recognition of neglect of the relationship on both sides. The importance of the suicide attempter acknowledging the hurt of their partner and making concerted efforts to reassure and repair the relationship, as well as the participant's willingness to accept this reassurance, is paramount. The function of forgiveness is ultimately to enhance healing within the relationship but it can also positively impact the well-being of the forgiver, in this case the partner of the individual who made the attempt on their life.

The final stage, 'the tree that bears new fruit', highlights the implications of new personal insights and insights about one's partner for growth that transcends the poison of the infidelity. This entails taking risks through sharing of intense emotions and unmet needs in order to cultivate a 'relationship culture' that espouses shared values and goals for the future.

A key component of this three-stage model is the integration of a mindfulness philosophy throughout the process. Modelling non-judgemental awareness on the part of the therapist can facilitate the couple in moving beyond intense negative feelings and remaining open to the lived experience of their partner. Taking a mindfulness approach during the therapeutic process could potentially support the therapist/clinician in moving beyond issues of counter-transference relating to family of origin or the therapist's own relationship history, as well as assumptions and prejudices about betrayal or attempted suicide.

Implications for policy

The main findings of this study would suggest that current policy and procedure surrounding the management of care post-suicide attempt need to take into account the welfare of the partner as well as that of the individual who has made the suicide attempt. Taking a Heideggerian perspective, an individual in an established meaningful relationship who makes a suicide attempt is a 'person-in-context'. A significant part of their context is their partner who will probably be traumatized either on hearing about the attempt or as a result of being directly exposed to it. They may also initially experience ambiguous loss and attachment injury, thereby shattering their assumptive world and creating great uncertainty about their past, present, and future circumstances. Current policy, however, operates upon the assumption that partners are in an immediate position to undertake the substantial caregiver role that is required once a suicidal individual is discharged from medical or other in-patient care. It is recommended that policy and procedure take a systems approach to the management of suicide attempters in established relationships. Interventions such as psycho-education for partners aimed at normalizing the personal impact for them, and a referral pathway for both individual and couples therapy, would increase the chances of recovery for both partner *and* the suicide attempter.

A number of systematic reviews of help-seeking behaviour in relatives of young people who have self-harmed, for example, have highlighted that they tend to be slow to seek out support due to feelings of guilt and/or shame and for fear of being negatively judged (National Institute for Health and Care Excellence, 2012; Curtis *et al.*, 2018). Greater public awareness of the impact on relatives, particularly partners, would serve to inform both primary and secondary care staff regarding tailored intervention. It would also serve to reduce stigma, thereby prompting partners to engage social support in order to sustain them during this traumatic time. As per Tedeschi and Calhoun (2004), disclosure within a supportive group environment might also increase the possibility for post-traumatic growth.

In the UK, many NHS Trusts have a well-established 'care programme approach' or CPA (Rethink Mental Illness, 2021) designed specifically to coordinate secondary mental health services for individuals exhibiting mental health problems, including suicide attempts. In Ireland, a National Clinical Programme for the assessment and management of patients presenting to emergency departments following self-harm began roll-out across the country in December 2014. This strategy was in direct response to the high numbers of individuals presenting to hospital emergency departments having self-harmed, over 11,000 in 2014 alone

(Wrigley, Jennings, MacHale and Cassidy, 2017). Neither the CPA nor the National Clinical Programme acknowledges the psychological and emotional well-being for partners of attempters, both in their own right and as a means of increasing the likelihood of recovery for suicide attempters. In fact the National Clinical Programme considers the carer or family member solely as a 'bridging strategy' to ensure that the patient will attend his or her 'next care' appointment following discharge from hospital. One of the goals cited by the National Clinical Programme for 2019/2020 was for the National Implementation Advisory Group to revise the model of care (Health Service Executive, 2021). It is my view that the model of care needs to broaden its scope beyond the suicide attempter to include care of the partner in the immediate aftermath of the attempt, rather than perpetuate an outdated assumption that a partner will be physically, emotionally, and spiritually untouched by this event and will, in fact, have the capacity, motivation, and desire to fully integrate it as simply part of the journey of their relationship. They may or may not be able to do this, but this needs to be assessed for, rather than conceptualized as a 'fait accompli'. Their lived experience needs to be respected *as well as* the lived experience of the individual who has attempted suicide. I am pleased, however, that this is now also being viewed as a priority at national level with the updated Model of Care due to be released in 2021, recognizing the need to provide concomitant support to family members (personal communication with the National Lead Dr. Anne Jeffers, April 2021).

Implications for primary care and psychotherapy practice

Although the immediate welfare of the suicidal individual is and should be the priority of first responders such as doctors, nurses, and psychiatrists, the findings of this study indicate that it is paramount that the vulnerability of the partner be acknowledged by these professionals as well as those providing longer-term secondary care such as psychotherapists. Partners are likely to display very individual responses to the attempted suicide and, therefore, need to be met by staff with sensitivity and respect. The findings of this study provide the foundations for a model of psychotherapeutic intervention aimed at partners of individuals who have attempted suicide. The model would serve as a means of highlighting the experience for partners as traumatic, normalize feelings associated with it including socially unsanctioned 'shadow side' feelings, recognize the phenomenon for partners as a loss that is ambiguous in nature, explore resilience building and finding meaning in the midst of ambiguous loss and boundary ambiguity, and aid partners in recognizing feelings of betrayal as a potential opportunity for relationship transformation. In addition, although growth in the wake of trauma and loss is not inevitable, psychotherapists can support partners in 'normalizing' the notion that growth can and does occur (Smith, Joseph and Das Nair, 2011).

A significant aspect of this model is psycho-educational in approach. Rather than immediately offering guidelines on providing care to the suicide attempter, partners first need to be educated about the nature of trauma and the potential for a delayed reaction. Partners should be provided with an opportunity to express feelings such as shock, confusion, fear, guilt, and helplessness. Significantly, this study has found that partners should be invited to explore potential 'shadow side' feelings such as disappointment, anger, resentment, abandonment, betrayal and violation of trust with a view to normalizing them. In addition, psychotherapists can provide insight into the complex relationship between trauma and compassion fatigue that is likely to manifest as part of a partner's lived experience.

The partner's level of resilience, that is, the degree to which they can sustain themselves through this life crisis and recover from it, should also be assessed. It may prove disadvantageous to assume that a partner will be physically and psychologically capable of coping with the suicide attempter returning to the family home immediately following discharge from hospital. Discharging patients into the care of those who are neither capable nor motivated to offer care to their suicidal partner may actually exacerbate the situation for both parties concerned. Recall the finding that individuals are at greater risk of suicide after discharge from hospital particularly within the first month (Deisenhammer *et al.*, 2007). It is paramount, therefore, that the partner's psychological and emotional well-being be given due consideration and that *both* partners receive ongoing aftercare following discharge. In the case where an individual receives in-patient care within a psychiatric facility, ongoing assessment and intervention for both partners should be considered, to include individual and couple psychotherapeutic input.

A variable known as 'event centrality' has been suggested as a significant predictor of both negative and positive trauma outcomes (Groleau Calhoun, Cann and Tedeschi, 2013). Event centrality can be described as 'the extent an event has been incorporated into an individual's [sense of self and] identity' (Schuettler and Boals, 2011, p. 184). Consequently, if 'centrality' occurred to a high degree for participants following the attempted suicide of their partners, then factors such as coping (avoidant/problem-focused) and perspective-taking (negative/ positive) may have influenced the direction the trauma took. Groleau *et al.* (2013) champion the view that psychotherapists should begin to pay attention to event centrality following a potentially traumatic experience.

Implications for psychotherapy training

Trainee psychotherapists need to be made aware about snap-shot assigning of the care-giver role to partners. Rather than being viewed in a one-dimensional way, partners need to be met by psychotherapists as multi-dimensional human beings whose assumptions about their world have just been shattered. Furthermore, by taking a systems approach and ensuring the welfare of partners, both partners are likely to fare better long term. Psychotherapists need also to make themselves aware of trauma with a small 't' rather than overreliance on diagnostic criteria for PTSD or capital 'T'. Training on ambiguous loss and interventions for building resilience and finding meaning, attachment injury and injury as opportunity for transformation, and recognizing and reinforcing signs of post-traumatic growth are all aspects of this phenomenon that could comprise continuous professional development for psychotherapists. In addition, emergency department personnel, particularly nurses, as well as mental health practitioners including psychologists, psychiatrists, and psychotherapists could benefit from reconfiguring the lived experience for partners as traumatic, and offer triage and an appropriate referral pathway for *both* partners.

Theoretical transferability

The recorded stories of participants were analyzed using a qualitative methodology known as Interpretive Phenomenological Analysis or IPA (Smith *et al.*, 2009). This methodology emphasizes the idiographic and the fact that accounts need to be viewed as local and always within a particular context. Smith, Flowers and Larkin (2009) advocate thinking 'in terms of theoretical transferability rather than empirical generalizability' (p. 51). Examples of groups within a similar context to the phenomenon of partner impact following attempted suicide, who may theoretically have also experienced both adverse and positive transformations, are 'significant others', such as parents or siblings who may also experience trauma, ambiguous loss, attachment injury, and post-traumatic growth. Other groups are individuals whose partners experience adverse outcomes from choosing to engage in behaviours involving risk such as substance misuse; physical disability or acquired brain injury following dangerous sports, serious financial debt due to gambling, and relationship transgressions such as infidelity.

Implications for future research

This study is the first of its kind to place full emphasis on the personal lived experience of individuals following the suicide attempt of their partner. Future studies could conduct additional in-depth analyses of the personal impact on partners in order to further explicate this phenomenon.

Further research could explore the complex phenomenon of concomitant primary and secondary (compassion fatigue) traumatic stress that was found within the present study, and explore this manifestation among other significant others or groups within a similar context.

The average time since the suicide attempt in the present study was 10.5 years. Further research might take a temporal approach to the lived experience for partners ranging from short to long term since the attempt in order to gain insight into any variance in coping, adjustment, and outlook over time.

The present study captured the experience of just one man. It may be illuminating to explore convergence and divergence between the sexes. Further studies in this area could also ascertain the attitudes of first responders or representatives of secondary mental health services to partners of those who attempt suicide in order to highlight their expectations of them.

In the context of relationships, future research could invite both partners to explore their lived experience pre- and post-suicide attempt in order to illuminate both risk and protective factors in the context of suicide.

Based on the findings of the current study, future research could administer psychometric tests on traumatic stress, ambiguous loss, boundary ambiguity, attachment injury and post-traumatic growth in order to ascertain the extent of theoretical generalisability.

Conclusion

The main finding of this study suggests that the impact of a individual's suicide attempt is transformational for partners, with both negative and positive trajectories. Adverse transformation occurred for participants as a result of the trauma suffered by them during this life-changing experience. Transformations, both positive and negative, continued during the complex adjustment, as they navigated through the intricacies of blame and self-preservation. The experience ultimately has left a legacy that has also been transformative in various ways, bringing to the surface what lay beneath and embracing new growth. Transformation was explored through the lens of trauma theory, ambiguous loss theory and boundary ambiguity, attachment theory, and post-traumatic growth.

I hope that these research findings and implications for practice, policy, training and future directions have been 'transformative' for the reader in challenging their view of the personal impact on partners as profound and far-reaching. One important outcome of this study, therefore, may be to champion a reframing of partners from solely care-givers, to persons in their own right.

REFERENCES

Aldwin, C.M. (1994). *Stress, Coping, and Development*. New York: Guilford.

American Foundation for Suicide Prevention (2021). Suicide Statistics. Available from: https://afsp.org/suicide-statistics (accessed 9 April 2021).

American Psychiatric Association (2013). *Diagnostic and Statistical Manual of Mental Disorders*, 5th edn. Arlington, VA: American Psychiatric Association.

Atkinson, L. (1997). 'Attachment and psychopathology: from laboratory to clinic', in L. Atkinson and K.J. Zucker (eds), *Attachment and Psychopathology*. New York: Guilford Press, pp. 3–16.

Attig, T. (2004). 'Disenfranchised grief revisited: discounting hope and love'. *Omega*, 49, 197–215.

Beautrais, A.L. (2004). *Support for Families, Whanau and Significant Others after a Suicide Attempt: A Literature Review and Synthesis of Evidence*. Christchurch: Christchurch School of Medicine and Health Sciences.

Boss, P.G. (1980). 'Normative family stress: family boundary changes across the life-span'. *Family Relations*, 29(4), 17–22.

Boss, P. (1987). 'Family stress', in M.B. Sussman and S.K. Steinmetz (eds), *Handbook of Marriage and Family*. New York: Plenum, pp. 695–723.

Boss, P. (1999). *Ambiguous Loss: Learning to Live with Unresolved Grief*. London: Harvard University Press.

Boss, P. (2004). 'Ambiguous loss research, theory, and practice: reflections after 9/11'. *Journal of Marriage and Family*, 66(3), 551–566. Available from: www.jstor.org/stable/3600212 (accessed 6 February 2021).

Boss, P. (2006). *Loss, Trauma, and Resilience: Therapeutic Work with Ambiguous Loss*. New York: Norton.

Boss, P. (2007). 'Ambiguous loss theory: challenges for scholars and practitioners'. *Family Relations*, 56(2), 105–111.

Boss, P. (2010). 'The trauma and complicated grief of ambiguous loss'. *Pastoral Psychology*, 59(2), 137–145.

Boss, P. (2016). The Context and Process of Theory Development: The Story of Ambiguous Loss. *Journal of Family Theory & Review*, 8: 269-286. https://doi.org/10.1111/jftr.12152

Boss, P. (2018). Building resilience: The example of ambiguous loss. In B. Huppertz (Ed.,) *Approaches to psychic trauma:Theory and practice* (pp. 91-105). Lanham, MD: Rowman & Littlefield.

Boss, P.G., Greenberg, J.R. and Pearce-McCall, D. (1990). 'Measurement of boundary ambiguity in families'. *Station Bulletin*, 593–1990, Minnesota Agricultural Experiment Station, University of Minnesota.

Boss, P., Pearce-McCall, D. and Greenberg, J. (1987). 'Normative loss in mid-life families: rural, urban, and gender differences'. *Family Relations*, 36, 437–443.

Bowlby, J. (1969). *Attachment and Loss*. Vol.1. *Attachment*. New York: Basic.

Bowlby, J. (1979). *The Making and Breaking of Affectional Bonds*. London: Tavistock.

Bowlby, J. (1988). *A Secure Base*. New York: Basic.

Bray, P. (2013). 'Bereavement and transformation: a psycho-spiritual and post-traumatic growth perspective'. *Journal of Religion and Health*, 52(3), 890–903.

Brewin, C.R., Andrews, B. and Valentine, J.D. (2000). 'Meta-analysis of risk factors for posttraumatic stress disorder in trauma-exposed adults'. *Journal of Consulting and Clinical Psychology*, 68(5), 748–766.

Calhoun, L. G. and Tedeschi, R. G. (1998). 'Posttraumatic growth: future directions', in R.G. Tedeschi, C.L. Park and L.G. Calhoun (eds), *Postraumatic Growth: Positive Change in the Aftermath of Crisis*. Mahwah, NJ: Lawrence Erlbaum Associates, pp. 215¬238.

Carroll, J.S., Olson, C.D. and Buckmiller, N. (2007). 'Family boundary ambiguity: a 30-year review of theory, research, and measurement'. *Family Relations*, 56(2), 210–230.

Curtis, S., Thorn, P., McRoberts, A., Hetrick, S., Rice, S. and Robinson, J. (2018). 'Caring for young people who self-harm: a review of perspectives from families and young people'. *International Journal of Environmental Research and Public Health*, 15(5), 950. Available from: https://doi.org/10.3390/ijerph15050950 (accessed 21 February 2021).

Dahl, C.M. and Boss, P. (2020). Ambiguous Loss. In *The Handbook of Systemic Family Therapy* (eds K.S. Wampler, M. Rastogi and R. Singh). https://doi.org/10.1002/9781119788409.ch6

Daszko, M. and Sheinberg, S. (2017). *Survival is Optional: Only Leaders with New Knowledge can Lead the Transformation* Available from: https://static1.squarespace.com/static/5912a7a5725e2534f1acb123/t/59234bc72e69cfef729 2c881/1495485386266/TRANSFORMATION-+A+DEFINITIO N%2C+THEORY%2C+AND+THE+CHALLENGES+TO+TRA NSFORMING.pdf (accessed 6 February 2021).

Deisenhammer, E.A., Huber, M., Kemmler, G, Weiss, E. M. and Hinterhuber, H. (2007). 'Psychiatric hospitalizations during the last 12 months before suicide'. *General Hospital Psychiatry*, 29(1), 63–65.

Doka, K. (2002). *Disenfranchized Grief: New Directions, Challenges, and Strategies for Practice*. Champaign, IL: Research Press.

Dupree, W.J., White, M.B., Shoup Olsen, C. and Lafleur, C.T. (2007). 'Infidelity treatment patterns: a practice-based evidence approach'. *American Journal of Family Therapy*, 35(4), 327–347.

Ebert, B. (2010). *Transformation in Psychotherapy. ACBS World Conference, Reno*. Available from: http://contextualscience.org/system/files/Transformation%20 in%20Psychotherapy.ppt (accessed 13 February 2021).

Feeney, J.A. (2004). 'Hurt feelings in couple relationships: towards integrative models of the negative effects of hurtful events'. *Journal of Social and Personal Relationships*, 21(4), 487–508.

Feeney, J.A. (2005). 'Hurt feelings in couple relationships: exploring the role of attachment and perceptions of personal injury'. *Personal Relationships*, 12(2), 253–271.

Feilgeson, C. (1993). Personality death, object loss, and the uncanny. International Journal of Psychoanalysis, 74(2), 331–345.

Figley, C.R. (ed.) (1995). *Compassion Fatigue: Coping with Secondary Traumatic Stress Disorder in those who Treat the Traumatized*. New York: Routledge.

Fosha, D. (2006). Quantum transformation in trauma and treatment: traversing the crisis of healing change. *Journal of Clinical Psychology: In Session*, 62(5), 569-–583.

Grof, S. (2000). *The Psychology of The Future*. Albany, NY: New York Press.

Groleau, J.M., Calhoun, L.G., Cann, A. and Tedeshi, R.G. (2013). 'The role of centrality of events in posttraumatic distress and posttraumatic growth'. *Psychological Trauma: Theory, Research, Practice, and Policy*, 5(5), 477–483.

Gustafsson, L. (1999). '... but no one loves me. A study of suicide in Västerbotten'. *Nordic Journal of Psychiatry*, 53(5), 390–391.

Harris, R. A. (1966). 'Factors related to continued suicidal behaviour in dyadic relationships'. *Nursing Research*, 15(1), pp. 72–75.

Harvey, L. (2019). *Social Research Glossary*. Quality Research International. Available from: www.qualityresearchinternational. com/socialresearch (accessed 6 February 2021).

Health Service Executive (2021). *Self Harm Presentation to ED*. Available from: www.hse.ie/eng/about/who/cspd/ncps/mental-health/self-harm (accessed 13 February 2021).

Hvidkjær, K.L., Ranning, A., Madsen, T., Feischer, E., Eckardt, J.P., Hjorthøj, C., Cerel, J. and Nordentoft, M. (2020). 'People exposed to suicide attempts: frequency, impact, and the support received'. *Suicide and Life-Threatening Behavior*. Available from: https://doi.org/10.1111/sltb.12720 (accessed: 28 March 2021).

Irish Health (2021). *Fibromyalgia*. Available from: www.irishhealth. com/article.html?con=384 (accessed 06 February 2021).

Janoff-Bullman, R. (1992). *Shattered Assumptions: Towards a New Psychology of Trauma*. New York: The Free Press.

Johnson, S.M. (1996). *The Practice of Emotionally Focused Marital Therapy: Creating Connection*. Philadelphia, PA: Brunner/Mazel.

Johnson, S.M., Makinen, J.A. and Millikin, J.W. (2001). 'Attachment injuries in couple relationships: a new perspective on impasses in couples therapy'. *Journal of Marital and Family Therapy*, 27(2), 145–155.

Joseph, S. and Linley, P.A. (2005). 'Positive adjustment to threatening events: an organismic valuing theory of growth through adversity'. *Review of General Psychology*, 9(3), 262–280.

Juel, A., Berring, L.L., Hybholt, L., Erlangsen, A., Larsen, E.R. and Buus, N. (2020). 'Relatives' experiences of providing care for individuals with suicidal behaviour conceptualized as a moral career: A meta-ethnographic study'. *International Journal of Nursing Studies*, 113. Available from: https://doi.org/10.1016/j. ijnurstu.2020.103793 (accessed: 28 March 2021).

Laplanche, J. (1976). *Life and Death in Psychoanalysis*. Baltimore, MD: Johns Hopkin's University Press.

Landau, J. and Hissett, J. (2008). 'Mild traumatic brain injury: impact on identity and ambiguous loss in the family'. *Families, Systems, & Health, 26(1), 69–85.*

Leary, M.R. (2001). 'Toward a conceptualization of interpersonal rejection', in M. R. Leary (ed.), *Interpersonal Rejection.* New York: Oxford Press, pp. 3–20.

Leenaars, A.A. (2010). Review: Edwin S. Shneidman on suicide. *Suicidology-Online*, 1, 5–18. https://pdf4pro.com/amp/view/edwin-s-shneidman-on-suicide-2135af.html (accessed 14 July 2021).

McLaughlin, C., McGowan, I., Kernohan, G. and O'Neill, S. (2016). 'The unmet support needs of family members caring for a suicidal person'. *Journal of Mental Health*, 25(3), 212–216. Available from: DOI:10.3109/09638237.2015.1101421 (accessed 28 March 2021).

Magne-Ingvar, U. and Öjehagen, A. (1999a). 'Significant others of suicide attempters: their views at the time of the acute psychiatric consultation'. *Social Psychiatry and Psychiatric Epidemiology*, 34, 73–79.

Magne-Ingvar, U. and Öjehagen, A. (1999b). 'One-year follow-up of significant others of suicide attempters'. *Social Psychiatry and Psychiatric Epidemiology*, 34, 470–476.

Mälkki, K. (2012). 'Rethinking disorienting dilemmas within real-life crises: the role of reflection in negotiating emotionally chaotic experiences'. *Adult Education Quarterly*, 62(3), 207–229.

McGann, V. L., Sands, D. C. & Gutin, N. (in press) Grief following suicide. In H. L. Servaty-Seib & H. S. Chapple (Eds.). *Handbook of Thanatology* (3rd edition). Association for Death Education and Counseling.

Mezirow, J. (1990). *Fostering Critical Reflection in Adulthood.* Oxford: Jossey-Bass.

Moon, P.J. (2011). 'Bereaved elders: transformative learning in late life'. *Adult Education Quarterly*, 61(1), 22 –39.

National Institute for Health and Clinical Excellence (2012). *Self-Harm: The NICE Guideline on Longer-Term Management.* Leicester: British Psychological Society and The Royal College of Psychiatrists.

National Office for Suicide Prevention (2021). *Briefing on CSO Suicide Figures 18th January 2021.* Available from: www.hse.ie/eng/services/list/4/mental-health-services/connecting-for-life/publications/nosp-briefing-jan-2021.pdf (accessed 06 February 2021).

Neimeyer, R.A. (2000). *Lessons of Loss: A Guide to Coping*. Clayton South: Australian Centre for Grief Education.

Neimeyer, R. A., & Sands, D. C. (2017) Meaning Reconstruction. In Grad, O. J., Andriessen, K., Krysinska, K., (Eds.), *Postvention in Action: The international handbook of suicide bereavement support*. Gottingen/Boston, Hoegrefe.

O'Brien, M. (2007). 'Ambiguous loss in families of children with autism spectrum disorders'. *Family Relations*, 56(2), 135–146.

Office for National Statistics (2020). Suicides in England and Wales: 2019 Registrations. Available from: www.ons.gov.uk/peoplepopulationandcommunity/birthsdeathsandmarriages/deaths/bulletins/suicidesintheunitedkingdom/2019registrations#:~:text=In%20total%20of,(10.5%20deaths%20per%20100%2C000) (accessed 06 February 2021).

Östman, M. and Kjellin, L. (2002). 'Stigma by association: psychological factors in relatives of people with mental illness'. *British Journal of Psychiatry*, 181, 494–498.

Östman, M., Wallsten, T. and Kjellin, L. (2005). 'Family burden and relative's participation in psychiatric care: are the patient's diagnosis and the relation to the patient of importance?' *International Journal of Social Psychiatry*, 51(4), 291–301.

Ozer, E. J., Best, S. R., Lipsey, T. L. and Weiss, D. S. (2008). 'Predictors of posttraumatic stress disorder and symptoms in adults: a meta-analysis'. *Psychological Trauma: Theory, Research, Practice, and Policy*, S(1), 3–36.

Padmanathan, P., Biddle, L., Hall, K., Scowcroft, E., Nielsen, E. and Knipe, D. (2019). 'Language use and suicide: An online cross-sectional survey'. *PLOS ONE* 14(6), e0217473. Available from: https://doi.org/10.1371/journal.pone.0217473 (accessed 6 February 2021).

Popadiuk, N. (2005). 'Family support: SAFER's concerned other program'. *Visions Journal*, 2(7), 37–38.

Rapoport, R. (1963). 'Normal crises, family structure, and mental health'. *Family Process*, 2(1), 68--80.

Rethink Mental Illness (2021). *Care Programme Approach* (CPA). Available from: www.rethink.org/advice-and-information/living-with-mental-illness/treatment-and-support/care-programme-approach-cpa/ (accessed 13 February 2021).

Sands, D. (2009). 'A tripartite model of suicide grief: meaning-making and the relationship with the deceased'. *Grief Matters: The Australian Journal of Grief and Bereavement*, 12(1), 10–17.

Sands, D. and Tennant, M. (2010). 'Transformative learning in the context of suicide bereavement'. *Adult Education Quarterly*, 60(2), 99–121.

Schuettler, D. and Boals, A. (2011). 'The path to posttraumatic growth versus posttraumatic stress disorder: contributions of event centrality and coping'. *Journal of Loss and Trauma*, 16, 180–194.

Segerstrom, S.C. and Miller, G.E. (2004). 'Psychological stress and the human immune system: a meta-analytic study of 30 years of inquiry'. *Psychological Bulletin*, 130(4), 601–630.

Smith, J.A., Flowers, P. and Larkin, M. (2009). *Interpretative Phenomenological Analysis: Theory, Method and Research*. London: Sage.

Smith, A., Joseph, S. and Das Nair, R. (2011). 'An interpretative phenomenological analysis of posttraumatic growth in adults bereaved by suicide'. *Journal of Loss and Trauma: International Perspectives on Stress & Coping*, 16(5), 413–430.

Stengel, E. (1956). 'The social effects of attempted suicide'. *Canadian Medical Association Journal*, 74, 116–120.

Sun, F.K., Long, A., Huang, X.Y. and Huang, H.M. (2008). 'Family care of Taiwanese patients who had attempted suicide: a grounded theory study'. *Journal of Advanced Nursing*, 62 (1), 53–61.

Sun, F.K., Long, A., Huang, J.Y. and Chiang, C.Y. (2009). 'A grounded theory study of action/interaction strategies used when Taiwanese families provide care for formerly suicidal patients'. *Public Health Nursing*, 26(6), 543–552.

Sun, F.K., Chiang, C.Y., Lin, Y.H. and Chen, T.B. (2013). 'Short-term effects of a suicide education intervention for family caregivers of people who are suicidal'. *Journal of Clinical Nursing*, 23, 91–102.

Sun, F.K., Long, A., Tsao, L.I. and Huang, H.M. (2014). 'The healing process following a suicide attempt: context and intervening conditions'. *Archives of Psychiatric Nursing*, 28, 55–61.

Talseth, A.G., Gilje, F. and Norberg, A. (2001). 'Being met – a passageway to hope for relatives of patients at risk of committing suicide: a phenomenological hermeneutic study'. *Archives of Psychiatric Nursing*, 15 (6), 249–256.

Taylor, E.W. (2007). 'An update on transformative learning theory:

a critical review of the empirical research (1999-2005)'. *International Journal of Lifelong Education*, 26(2), 173–191.

Taylor, S. (2012). 'Transformation through suffering: a study of individuals who have experienced positive transformation following periods of intense turmoil'. *Journal of Humanistic Psychology*, 52(1), 30–52.

Tedeschi, R.G. and Calhoun, L.G. (2004). 'Posttraumatic growth: conceptual foundations and empirical evidence'. *Psychological Inquiry*, 15(1), 1–18.

Tierney, M. (2011). 'As one person per day commits suicide, Console is needed more than ever'. *Galway Advertiser* Ireland, 10 February. Available from: www.advertiser.ie/galway/article/36326 (accessed 22 May 2021).

Vangelisti, A.L. (2001). 'Making sense of hurtful interactions in close relationships', in V. Manusov and J.H. Harvey (Eds), *Attribution, Communication Behavior, and Close Relationships*. New York: Cambridge University Press, pp. 38–58.

Warren, J.A., Morgan, M.M., Williams, S.L. and Mansfield, T.L. (2008). 'The poisoned tree: infidelity as opportunity for transformation'. *The Family Journal*, 16, 351–358.

Wolk-Wasserman, D. (1986). 'Suicidal communication of persons attempting suicide and responses of significant others'. *Acta Psychiatrica Scandinavica*, 73, 481–499.

Worden, J.W. (2009). *Grief Counselling and Grief Therapy: A Handbook for the Mental Health Practitioner*, 4th edn. NY: Springer.

World Health Organization (1992). *The ICD-10 Classification of Mental and Behavioural Disorders: Clinical Descriptions and Diagnostic Guidelines*. Geneva: World Health Organization.

World Health Organization: Mental and Behavioural Disorders Team (1999). *Figures and Facts about Suicide*. Geneva: World Health Organization. https://apps.who.int/iris/handle/10665/66097

World Health Organization (2021). *Background of SUPRE. Prevention of Suicidal Behaviours: A Task for All*. Available from: www.who.int/mental_health/prevention/suicide/background/en/ (accessed 09 April 2021).

Wrigley, M., Jennings, R., MacHale, S. and Cassidy, E. (2017). 'Assessment and management of self harm in emergency departments in Ireland: The national clinical programme'. *International Journal of Integrated Care*, 17(5), A312. DOI. http://doi.org/10.5334/ijic.3629 (accessed 06 February 2021).

Zautra, A.J., Hall, J.S. and Murray, K.E. (2010). 'Resilience: a new definition of health for people and communities' in J.W. Reich, A.J. Zautra and J.S. Hall, (eds), *Handbook of Adult Resilience*. New York: Guilford Press, pp. 3-32.

INDEX